BUTCHERED BY "HEALTHCARE"

WHAT TO DO ABOUT DOCTORS, BIG PHARMA, AND CORRUPT GOVERNMENT RUINING YOUR HEALTH AND MEDICAL CARE

ROBERT YOHO, MD

10/20
FOR MY FAVORITE
GIRL, VIV.

— ROBERT

10/20

For my FAVORITE

girl! ♥.

—Robert

PRAISE

You are to be commended for tackling an impossible subject. The core premise of the book is on point and timely. The metaphors and analogies are brilliant. I loved your description of statistics—relative versus absolute risk. The writing is excellent.

— JEFF SEGAL, MD, JD

A powerful attack on the status quo. You didn't pull any punches. I think the drug companies might put out a hit on you. The anecdotes and references provide an extra layering of depth to the conclusions. America's health care system does three things very well: make money, make money, and make money. And if along the way some patients get better....well bravo!

— MIKE STEELE, RN, RETIRED FROM A VETERANS ADMINISTRATION HOSPITAL

Fascinating… I read your book in a few days. It is lucid and readable. You share some of the same concerns I have had during my medical career. I think the system is so badly corrupted it is going to need to be demolished and replaced de novo. It is founded on the greedy self-interests of

numerous competing groups… Unbridled capitalism has no place in healthcare.

— Neal Handel, MD, West Hollywood, CA

The most important message in this book is that much of medicine is questionable theory presented as indisputable fact.

— Mira de Vries, metzelf.nl, Association for Medical and Therapeutic Self-Determination

At first blush, this book could be called a piece of investigative science journalism, but that would presuppose that the information is difficult to find. Rather, this information is open for all to see, yet we ignore it for political or personal reasons. Dr. Yoho's book is a well written, all-encompassing wake-up call for our dysfunctional and corrupt healthcare system. I hope it will also motivate individuals to take more responsibility for their own health.

— Paul Johnson, D.O.

AUTHOR'S NOTE

HOW YOU CAN SURVIVE "HEALTHCARE," THE LARGEST AND MOST CORRUPT INDUSTRY IN AMERICA.

> ✪ *Learn what works.* ✪ *See through the lies.* ✪ *Handle hospitals.* ✪ *Find trustworthy doctors.* ✪ *Master your drugs and quit them with confidence.* ✪ *Consider holistic medicine.*

Healthcare is the top cause of all our overdue debts and personal bankruptcy. Our medical spending per person is double that of other countries', but fully half the treatments are ineffective or harmful. Immense, predatory industries such as angioplasty and coronary artery bypass surgery victimize us. These procedures cause complications and deaths, but few patients survive even a day longer. Most back and endoscopic knee surgeries are equally worthless.

Seventy percent of us are on prescriptions, and 20 percent take over five. One in six uses psychiatric medicine, which commonly causes irreversible brain damage and premature death. Millions are now addicted to prescription opioids. Fifty-thousand people die each year from overdoses.

The FDA allows big Pharma to falsify the studies required to patent drugs. These corporations hire armies of ghostwriters to stuff websites and medical journal articles with marketing lies. Finding the truth is now nearly impossible. But all this gets overlooked as the companies pay billions of dollars in criminal settlements nearly every year.

Money short-circuits everyone's integrity, but there is an alternative. Patients and doctors can still prevail. Learn the system, and you can too.

For information, contact: RobertYohowriter@gmail.com

Robert Yoho MD Inc PC

PO Box 50007

Pasadena, California, 91115

Library of Congress Control Number: 2020915244

ISBN-13: Amazon: 978-1-7354857-0-6

978-1-7354857-3-7

paperback: 978-1-7354857-4-4

BISAC Subject Codes:

MED035000 MEDICAL / Health Care Delivery

HEA028000 HEALTH & FITNESS / Health Care Issues

BUS070170 BUSINESS & ECONOMICS / Industries / Healthcare

Disclaimers: I have no conflict of interest I can identify. I own no substantial healthcare stock, get paid nothing by corporate sources, and do not get paid by lawyers. I have no relationship or background with Scientology, which collectively hates psychiatry and psychiatric drugs.

If you are a patient, this book is no substitute for evaluation and treatment by a qualified, licensed health professional. The publisher and I do not recommend stopping, adding, or changing medication or therapy without consulting your doctor. You must look for a provider you trust and who is also willing to listen and learn—a rare beast. You should try to understand as much as you can about your health issues to help with the decisions.

As far as I am aware, the content here is current as of the date of publication. We expressly disclaim any liability arising directly or indirectly from the use or misuse of this information. By using this work, the user acknowledges and assumes responsibility for the accuracy or inaccuracy of the contents. No warranties are made by the copyright holder as to the accuracy of the material herein. By using this work, the user holds harmless and indemnifies Robert Yoho and Inverness Press from all liabilities generated from such use.

The stories here came from actual patients or doctors, who all gave permission. I sometimes changed their names and a few details to preserve privacy.

The statements and supporting arguments here are my opinions, based on expert sources: hundreds of professionals who have spent decades analyzing medical corruption. I am responsible for all errors, however.

❀ Created with Vellum

For the patients whose trust we betrayed. We have tortured them with useless or harmful surgeries, therapies, and medications. I tell the story hoping we can do better.

PART I
INTRODUCTION

CHAPTER 1

WHY WRITE ABOUT
HEALTHCARE CORRUPTION?

*Every surgeon carries within himself a small cemetery, where from
time to time he goes to pray—a place of bitterness and regret, where
he must look for an explanation for his failures.*

— *RENE LERICHE, LA PHILOSOPHIE DE LA CHIRURGIE,*
1951

IN THE SUMMER OF 2013, when I was 61, I had two women in
their 30s die in my surgical center. I sent them to the emergency room, but nothing worked. It was my place, so I was
responsible. It was the worst period of my life. I felt guilty
and was sleepless, and my wife thought we would have to
give up our practice.

I did not learn why it happened until the autopsy reports
came back six months later. One woman had an "embolus" of
fat blocking her lungs. This occurs unpredictably, and there is
no means to prevent it.

The second had a high local anesthetic blood level. We
inject this into fat to decrease pain, and after liposuction, we
sometimes transplant the fat back into breasts and buttocks.

This may have raised her levels and caused her death, but there was no way to be sure.

To occupy my mind, I started reading medicine twenty to thirty hours a week. My original training was as a generalist, but for decades I had studied only cosmetic surgery.

I began with the Prozac-class antidepressants, which I had prescribed since their invention. It stunned me to learn that they hardly worked and were often damaging. I read further and found that other psychiatric medications produce irreversible brain and health problems. Doctors have been trained to pass them out like jelly beans.

I learned that many drugs are given for wholly theoretical, even speculative benefits. Many are damaging. I consulted people for cosmetic surgery who were taking ten (10) of these at once. I began to see how medical corporations had done this to us.

MUCH

I read about back pain. Most of it goes away on its own, but doctors had been thoughtlessly prescribing opioid painkillers and turning many patients into struggling addicts. Back surgeries are the most expensive and some of the least effective procedures in all medical care, bar none. No one admits this even to themselves—not the surgeons, the hospital administrators, nor the surgical centers owners. The enormous profits short-circuit everybody's judgment.

I also realized that over the past three decades, younger and younger people had been getting heart disease, obesity, and diabetes. I wondered if healthcare, particularly medication use, might be the cause. I thought about Peter Van Etten's line, "In this insanity of healthcare, the patient always loses." I saw that we were breaking them on a medical torture-wheel.

———

THE AMOUNT of wealth thrown into American healthcare is astounding. Since the corporations took over, hospitals, drug

companies, and senior doctors on their payola are scrapping
for it like giant carp eating bread. We pay them handsomely
for anything they can slap a billing code on, and they dictate
every move according to profitability. Patient wellbeing is
now secondary. Healthcare quality—and our general health—
has deteriorated.

I have affluent peers, and some are not shy about it. A
gastroenterologist boasted in the doctors' lunchroom that he
puts diamonds on the fingers of his infant daughters. In 2004,
a cardiologist wearing a $3000 suit told me he "couldn't pay
his personal expenses" if he made less than $600,000 a year.
Nouveau riche posturing like this is usually accompanied by
stories about expensive, supposedly lifesaving treatments. I
always vaguely smelled a rat, but I was busy and never gave
it much thought.

As I continued to study, I realized that newer science
proved that many of the therapies these people were selling
were worthless. I wondered what profit their fancy cars or
high incomes could be for them if they did not put patients
first.

After a great deal of personal and professional reflection, I
decided to write about the whole medical-industrial calamity.
I understand I am a whistleblower, what it means, and what I
face. One of my source authors warned me I would lose my
medical license. In late 2019, I quit practicing and left the
melee. I can now say what I need to from outside the tent and
without conflicts of interest.

My story is not the narrative of *Wikipedia*, *WebMD*, or
other online sources. These are constantly being rewritten by
marketers. *Wiki* is the most reliable, but like the others, it is
under guerrilla attack by corporate ghostwriters. Most physicians disagree with me as well. When I shared my conclusions with them, most became resentful, cited their training,
and told me I was dead wrong. The few who know the story
are afraid to speak up.

Industry shills and people born yesterday say my tale is dated and claim everything has changed. They are right—it is not a new story. Since information remains concealed until drugs are off-patent, some of my references are ten to twenty years old. But they are only half-right: they are wrong about the change—the situation has become progressively worse.

Even though this history has been an open secret for decades, only an elite few understand the whole dysfunctional puzzle. You have the chance to join them, but the more you learn, the more it will break your heart.

For physicians, to practice effectively and ethically, they must understand what they face. Familiarity with these controversies is indispensable, even if you reject some conclusions. Your work will improve after you realize that doing less may produce better results.

Likewise, patients must learn about these issues to have the best chance of benefiting from healthcare. I share practical, little-known ways to deal with doctors and hospitals. You will also learn about health, sickness, and the limits of medicine. The more you know, the more confident you will be accepting —or in some cases, refusing care.

Despite my best efforts, I may be partly wrong. For example, statisticians are more optimistic than I am about the trifling improvements shown in large studies. You may also think you "know" about an area where I am mistaken, and that this destroys my credibility. For some cautious readers, what follows may even sound like a hostile, one-sided polemic.

So proceed with caution. If some disagreement kidnaps you and you quit reading, you will lose your chance to understand the ecosystem. Before feuding with me about a tree in this forest, scan at least the first dozen anecdotes. Money has poisoned our well, and this pattern establishes legitimacy even before you look at references. You need not swallow everything I serve up to believe that we are managing patients poorly.

The first step to deal with the situation, either as a doctor or a patient, is to learn the truth. This is also necessary for reform. By the end, you will understand the mess that has developed after we permitted industrialized medicine to snowball for thirty years.

Robert Yoho, MD, May 2020
DrYohowriter@gmail.com
Pasadena, CA

———

FOR POWER READERS

To learn this material, you do not need the three years that I took—you can get it in three hours. Approach it however you wish. Browse the headlines, read more carefully, or dive into thousands of references.

Warning: this is a genuine Greek tragedy. Some cannot [will not] tolerate going through it all at once. The *Patient Tips* chapters in between the others will give you breaks. Here, I share what you can do to help yourself and your families.

If you get bogged down, I suggest you at least finish the introductory section and scan the rest. Return for what you missed—it is all important.

Three "Blue's Clues"—practical heuristics—will help you decipher anything.

1) If you do not follow the reasoning, someone is likely lying to sell you something. You are as smart as the story-teller, so do not let them fool you. This applies to financial advisors and lawyers as well as to medical studies.

2) The updated Golden Rule is that those with the gold make the rules, so learning the source of funding explains a lot.

3) Controversy, confusion, and contradictory evidence

about small numbers *proves that whatever it is does not work.* Do not fall into the trap of believing that "reasonable people disagree" or "the science is developing."

Dragging politics into the healthcare debate inflames all sides. This makes problem-solving and cooperation impossible. The central issue is that over half of what we do is wasteful, ineffective, or harmful—this is our collective problem. Social support programs are also unrelated and are *not addressed here.*

I try to avoid political signaling, just as I avoid discussing religion or finances. Many of us have forgotten that polite company demands good manners, and some of us have become boors. Additionally, good doctors do not babble about these topics with patients because they are "boundary violations" that taint relationships and are prejudicial to proper care.

Not even China, whose leaders try to rewrite history, can hide from web crawlers. Although about ten percent of links disappear every year because of "link rot," virtually everything that was ever seen on the Web is still alive and well on the Wayback Machine Internet archive. Just copy the bad link (the web address at the top of the browser) and enter it at archive.org. Then look for the backed-up copies and select the date you want to view. You can also save any URL indefinitely for free at another of their pages. These are Internet superpowers that are handy to have in your bookmarks.

Blasting through certain paywalls is easy. *Sci-hub* is a "piracy" website based in Russia. It will get you some academic articles at no charge. Just copy the link into their browser. This is against the law, but some academics publicly thank them.

Journals are no better than the rest of the medical money-grubbers. Their paywalls price-gouge and impede scientific exchange. When you read *The Sins of the Journals'* chapter later, you will become angry enough that you will not feel guilty when you use sci-hub. Whether you pay for articles is a private matter between you, the journal, Sci-hub, and your maker.

About our relationship: I am distributing this book free for a limited time at this LINK. If you do not understand e-books, the support people there will help you download an app and start reading. If you haven't discovered Kindle or other ebook readers, you will find they are the easiest way to read—anything—and handily access references. Here is my website: DrYohoAuthor.com. Click this LINK for my author site on Amazon.

I answer all polite questions at DrYohoauthor@gmail.com. Email if you want me to speak to your group. Mailing address: P O Box 50007, Pasadena, CA, 91115. Website for my (former) cosmetic surgery career: DrYoho.com.

CHAPTER 2

I WAS WRONG ABOUT HEALTHCARE

*Wholly unprepared... we take the step into the afternoon of life;
worse still, we take this step with the false assumption that our
truths and ideals will serve as before. But we cannot live the
afternoon of life according to the program of life's morning—for
what was great in the morning will be little at evening, and what in
the morning was true will at evening have become a lie.*

— CARL JUNG

DOCTORS HELP PATIENTS, and they love us for it. We fix bones,
replace joints, cure killer infections, and control diabetes
with insulin. We use painless scans for diagnosis. Liver,
kidney, and heart transplants are now routine. Some
patients get cured of lymphomas, leukemia, Hodgkin's
disease, and testicular cancer. Lives are prolonged for
myeloma and amyloidosis. Vaccines have saved millions
worldwide.

We have complex technologies such as the heart bypass
machine and dialysis. We replace diseased heart valves with
artificial ones that work. Cardiologists permanently correct
irregular rhythms using techniques that would seem natural

on *Star Trek*. Other specialists gift infertile couples with children.

Despite this, many sources agree: for at least half of healthcare, the potential benefit does not outweigh the harm. For a lot of the rest, supporting evidence that it works is lacking. A review of over 5000 articles recommends against many of today's standard practices.

The list below introduces some of the topics in this book, the worst failures of healthcare, in rough order of wasted resources. The opioid disaster, now killing 50,000 people a year in the US, is not even in the top seven. I "knew" a lot because of my degrees and training, but I was wrong about many things.

1) Insurance.

What I thought: *health insurance protects us against disasters, just like fire insurance.*

The truth: Most of the $3.65 trillion in US medical spending (2018) is run through insurance companies before payment, which produces an insanity of wastefulness. These corporations extract fully a fifth—twenty dollars of every hundred!—of whatever they touch for their administration and profits, and they know that if total spending goes up, they get more money.

After the insurance layer has taken its share, only 75-80 percent remains for "providers" and suppliers. Every one of these has their own bloated overhead, which they must pay before patients get anything. Hospitals, for example, consume at least 25 percent more for internal expenses. This system creates outrageous total costs.

The smaller but more gloomy insurance story is the workers compensation system.

2) Hospitals.

What I thought: *hospitals are bureaucratic, but physicians supervise them to make people better.*

The truth: Although many people who work in hospitals

are idealistic, most of these corporations are ruthless pirates that are looting the patients who trust them. These companies pay or bully physicians to cooperate with their agendas.

Hospital costs are about a third of US healthcare. They spend ten to fifteen percent of their receipts just on coding, collections, and other methods to whip money out of the insurance companies.

3) Drugs and medical devices.

What I thought: *Idealistic scientists wearing white coats develop new miracle drugs and devices all the time.*

The truth: The pharmaceutical companies purposefully falsify the studies the FDA requires to patent medications, and the regulator turns a blind eye to it. Concealing negative studies that show little or no efficacy, such as was done with the antidepressants and the statin anti-cholesterol drugs, is just the start of their hoaxes. Because of practices like this, deciphering which medications work has become difficult. Many drugs are ineffective, and a lot are damaging. Some of the worst are the statins, the newer diabetes drugs, the osteoporosis drugs, the influenza vaccine, and the whole psychiatric pharmacy. These are all best-sellers.

The huge implant device industry plays the same games as the pharmaceutical companies and has fewer rules that force them to conduct proper studies.

Here is what I thought about generic drugs: *they are just about as good but cheaper than patent medicines, which are a rip-off.*

The truth: I was right; patent medicines are a rip-off. Generics are sometimes inactive or even contaminated, however. But they are now 90 percent of the American formulary because of patent drug price-gouging.

4) Journals and the academics of medicine:

What I thought: *If I studied hard, read journals, went to meetings, and listened rather than talking to my friends, I would become a better physician. Also, if I looked at Internet sources, I would quickly learn about any medical field.*

The truth: Doctors' information sources have been wrecked by corporations. We depend on journals, but their editors have been bought off. They print fraudulent studies containing purposefully confusing math developed by academics who are sponsored by corporations.

Patients' information sources, on the other hand, are advertising, "advocacy" groups, blogs written by industry, and wall-to-wall internet link-farms. They are all marketing in disguise and create anxiety and spread false information.

5) Mental Health.

What I thought: *psychiatrists have some strange ideas, but their drugs are effective and treat mental illness just like insulin helps diabetes.*

The truth: This is our most expensive and least effective medical sector. Informed commentators now call psychiatry a pseudo-science, and a substantial, credible group—besides Scientology—openly questions their theories and drugs.

Psychiatry is nearly divorced from even the flawed science advising the rest of medicine. The psychiatrists accept the most money from the pharmaceutical industry of any doctor group, which results in their ideas being the most contaminated. Their toxic medications might help a few sick people, but corporations promote them so heavily that one in six US citizens takes them. We mostly ignore the tragic consequences.

6) The heart industry.

What I thought: *cardiologists and heart surgeons have effective treatments for coronary artery disease.*

The truth: Invasive treatments for this are an immense but dismally ineffective industry. Sham surgery studies have now debunked stents, the tiny devices used to open coronary arteries. These might never work, depending on what you believe. The cardiologists understand the math yet continue placing them for the money.

Coronary artery bypass grafting surgery (CABG) is also useless or harmful. It immediately kills two to nine percent and gives long-term brain damage to a third. A few patients supposedly benefit: the three percent with severe blockage of their one-centimeter "left main" artery. For them, the studies show a five-year survival improvement of twenty (20) percent. But the operation is overwhelmingly performed for patients with other issues. These people suffer the complications with no chance of benefit.

Medications and lifestyle changes work better for coronary heart disease than these hazardous, invasive procedures.

7) Back pain.

What I thought: *prolonged recovery might be the rule after back injuries, but the treatments, including surgery, help.*

The truth: Unfortunately, our therapies are failures. Studies show every single one is an expensive, sometimes risky placebo. These include surgery, chiropractic, and the ultrasound and vibrators used by traditional physical therapists. Addictive opioid pain pills are prescribed long-term for chronic back pain, which is another disaster. Graduated exercise is the only treatment that helps these agonizing problems.

8) The opioid debacle.

What I thought: *the cause of the opioid disaster is physician overprescribing.*

The truth: Purdue Pharma and some other corporations late to the party were primarily responsible. Purdue marketed one of these drugs, OxyContin, to nearly anyone with a painful condition, claiming it was safe and not addictive. This started a trend that resulted in hundreds of thousands of deaths. Purdue declared bankruptcy in 2019, the first big pharmaceutical corporation ever dismantled by plaintiffs. Until this happened, the industry regarded legal problems merely as tolerable expenses, as their revenues were in the tens of billions.

9) Oncology or cancer treatment.

What I thought: *we have a lot of cures and the science is advancing rapidly.*

The truth: This is a heavily hyped sales pitch created by the industry. Cancer is the second leading cause of death after heart disease, but only a scant few treatments cure or even significantly prolong life. Although pain relief counts, extending life is the critical measure of success, and if the patient dies sooner of something else, it is a failure. Most of our toxic, over-advertised, extortionately priced treatments offer less than two months of prolonged survival.

Two-thirds of cancer doctors' income comes from retailing drugs, or rather getting "rebates" for selling them. This is legal for corporations, but it would likely be criminal fee-splitting if done between physicians. Whatever the legalities, manipulating patient care with financial incentives has over-whelming potential for abuse. This must be banned.

10) The amphetamine tragedy.

What I thought: *amphetamine abuse is mainly an issue for poor people in ghettos.*

The truth: As with opioids, the pharmaceutical companies' products are virtually identical to and produce the same disastrous effects as street drugs. Addicts use high doses, which make health destruction inevitable for this small group. Patients use lower doses, but prescriptions are so universal that this disaster is far more significant.

Corporations manipulate captive, well-paid psychiatrists to expand the indications for these drugs, despite the brain damage and behavior deterioration they cause. Nine percent of our children (a figure cited by the Centers for Disease Control) supposedly have "attention deficit hyperactivity disorder" (ADHD). Psychiatrists recommend medicating them. Many of our other kids get these medications from their friends.

The recent claim is that adults, including older people, also have an epidemic of ADHD, so they get prescriptions also. Some children now buy the drugs from their neighborhood senior citizen.

11) Mammograms.

What I thought: *mammograms save women from breast cancer.*

The truth: Mammograms used to check women without lumps or other indications are a waste of time, money, and emotional energy. Millions of these tests are performed each year, hundreds of thousands of them are positive or unclear, and untold women get repeated mammograms and ultrasound examinations to chase the findings. After this, biopsies and surgeries are done to evaluate and cut out the areas of concern.

This process is expensive, and each procedure is a little risky. But the math does not work—patients do not live longer after accounting for the hazards of the invasive procedures that ensue after a mammographic finding. We would be better off if the system only evaluated women with lumps they find themselves.

12) Colon cancer.

What I thought: *colonoscopy saves us from colon cancer.*

The truth: Colonoscopy for random patients looking for colon cancer has no benefit.

This tumor is the second most frequent cancer killer after lung cancer. US gastroenterologists look inside the colon to identify small cancers and pre-cancers before they spread. Since surgeons can often cure these in their early stages by cutting out a section of the colon, this screening program seems reasonable. But examining patients without symptoms or known disease does not increase the time they live.

13) Prostate cancer.

What I thought: *urologists save men from dying of prostate cancer by checking a blood test on everyone over a certain age.*

The truth: This does not work. The standard routine is to check the prostate-specific antigen (PSA) in the blood, and when it is high, to do painful biopsies. If cancer is seen, a removal operation called "radical prostatectomy" is often recommended. This commonly results in impotence and incontinence and saves no lives overall. Other therapies for the early stages of this cancer are also ineffective and damaging.

Even though about 75 percent of older men get prostate cancer before they die, it is only fatal in two percent. The tumor is usually inactive, and an aggressive approach does more harm than good.

14) Endoscopic knee surgery for arthritic knee and hip pain.

What I thought: *if my knees hurt, an endoscopic operation will help.*

The truth: Sham surgery studies compared patients who had this procedure versus those who only had incisions and anesthesia. There was no difference—the operation was a failure. The orthopedists know this, but they still perform this somewhat risky surgery. The costs in the US are $4 billion a year.

Whether you are a doctor or patient, the painful reality introduced here is running you over. The next two chapters explain how it all started and developed.

CHAPTER 3

HOW HEALTHCARE WAS RUINED

Cui Bono, the Latin phrase meaning "who benefits," says the motive for an act or event likely lies with the person who has something to gain.

HEALTHCARE COSTS STARTED GROWING NEARLY EXPONENTIALLY when social support programs and private insurance fueled it in the 1960s. US costs are now $3.65 trillion (2018), almost a fifth of our gross domestic product (GDP), and twice what other developed countries are paying per capita.

Our medical sector spends more than the total revenues of banking ($477 billion), oil and gas ($181 billion), and military ($600-800 billion). We spend more on healthcare than the next ten countries combined—more than France, Spain, China, Japan, Brazil, Germany, Italy, Canada, Australia, and the United Kingdom. Wealthy Singapore pays only a mid-single-figure percent of its GDP, and many others spend about ten percent.

Could the rest of the world be missing out? Are there advantages of more pills, surgeries, and doctor care? How is it even possible to spend this much money? Our academics know the answer: *excess healthcare makes providers money, but is a net harm for patients.*

All that spending attracted scammers and entrepreneurs, and they have pursued profits at the expense of patients. As a result, half of medical care is now ineffective, of unknown effectiveness, or harmful. Americans are less healthy and die sooner than people in other developed countries. Our average life expectancy is only 43rd in the world.

The excess spending damages our economy. Warren Buffett said healthcare is "The tapeworm of the American economy... the number 1 problem of America and of American business." Economist Peter Orszag agrees: "The United States' standing in the world depends on its success in constraining this healthcare cost explosion; unless it does, the country will eventually face a severe fiscal crisis or a crippling inability to invest in other areas."

———

HEALTHCARE RUINATION IN THREE STEPS

Note: Insurance companies, government, and corporate employers are "third-party payers." The first and second "parties" are the providers and the patients, who respectively give and receive care.

Step one: Easy money from insurance and government led to a gold-rush. Insurance companies administrate nearly the entire circus, producing astounding waste. These corporations skim off roughly 20 percent of all healthcare revenue (they oversee Medicare also) for their profits, lobbying, overhead, advertising, investor dividends, interior decorating, and stratospheric executive salaries. The remaining 80 percent goes to hospitals, doctors, and other providers so they can perform patient care. This is the "Medical Loss Ratio."

As a benchmark, in 2011, the Affordable Care Act (ACA) mandated these insurance expenses must be less than 20

percent. The insurance industry lobbied ferociously for more.
The ACA does not apply to companies which self-fund
healthcare coverage, where the percentage eaten by the insurance administration may be much higher. For example, in
2010, the Texas Blue Cross and Blue Shield expenses were 36
percent before they paid out anything for patients. Some say
Medicare has held its insurance administration close to 10
percent, but this is disputed, and others claim the costs per
person are even higher than for private insurance. Elisabeth
Rosenthal, in *An American Sickness* (2017), wrote that insurance administration costs now average 20 percent.

After insurance grabs its share, before anything goes for
patient care, providers spend another 15 to 30 percent on their
own internal profits, billing, advertising, and administrative
costs. To distribute all the money, a costly appendage of
codes, billing specialists, and supporting infrastructure
grew up.

This system produces astronomical expenses. A 2020
study in *Annals of Internal Medicine* by David Himmelstein
claims that in 2017, the total overhead was 31 percent. A *NY
Times* (2018) estimate by Austin Frakt was 30 percent. But
given the complexity and the figures above, these estimates
must be low.

Worse, ineffective services and outright frauds account for
at least half of all medical care costs. We barely recognize
these, so we do not count them as overhead.

When someone else pays, patients see it as a gift and
devalue it. When someone else pays, doctors have no qualms
about recommending the most expensive options—which are
often the most profitable for them. When someone else pays,
useless but lucrative tests and treatments become commonplace because there is no incentive to be sensible.

The result is that self-styled providers spend recklessly in
a dysfunctional, pseudo-capitalistic gold-rush. Nursing
homes, device manufacturers, hospital executives, and big

pharmaceutical firms are all at the feeding trough with the doctors. Care-givers and patients alike act as if they were at a buffet, eating until they get sick. This is free enterprise combined with remote payment: a large-scale, uniquely American disaster. It creates a savage cycle of escalating costs and declining standards.

Insurance companies waste much of their effort trying to keep rapacious providers from gulping down the whole pie. They must play games, such as arbitrarily switching billing codes or denying payments. Physicians in private practice who do not study the continually shifting reimbursement schemes make little money. Others who spend more time on billing than medical education make millions.

Higher and higher taxes and premiums pass the costs through to the rest of us. The system does not reward insurance companies to limit expenses because their share is a big slice right off of the top.

Step two: All that money caused corruption. The insurance system was conceived in good faith to supply vital care. But the gargantuan fountain of tax and insurance loot cannot be monitored.

Third-party payment combined with free-market profits encourages overuse of anything a provider can stick a bill on. Everyone is compensated by piecemeal and submits separate, competing charges, resulting in a frenzy of exaggerated and fraudulent invoices. The system allows payment for any covered medical treatment, so there is no upper limit on the total.

Since severe illnesses justify more reimbursement, hospitals and doctors do unnecessary lab tests and x-rays under the pretext that they suspect dangerous conditions. These create more bills and support invoices for extensive evaluations. Complicated, expensive treatments follow, which doctors order even if they are ineffective or damaging. Agatha Christie said, "When large sums of money are involved, it is advisable to trust nobody." She might have added, "Not even your doctor or hospital."

The Center for Responsive Politics reports that this industry, including doctors, spent $5.36 billion from 1998 to 2006 on Congressional lobbying. It was far more than the combined spending of defense and aerospace ($1.53 billion), plus oil and natural gas interests ($1.3 billion) during the same period.

These industries have promotional budgets like this because their money came from government payments, subsidies, or tax breaks—ultimately, the taxpayers. All of us fund this lobbying.

As I uncovered story after story of physicians' and industry's ethical perversions, I understood Cicero's maxim: "Nothing is so strongly fortified that it cannot be taken with money." Business people understand this, but physicians, who are trained more like academics, are able to pretend their behavior is kosher.

Step three: Ever since profit became the primary goal, patient welfare is neglected, and half of our care became ineffective or harmful. This is the worst of the three, but it is almost unrecognized.

A *Scientific American* article (2011) describes the failure: "We could accurately say, 'Half of what physicians do is wrong,' or 'Less than 20 percent of what physicians do has solid research to support it.' Although these claims sound absurd, they are solidly supported by research that is largely agreed upon by experts. Yet these claims are rarely discussed publicly. It would be political suicide…"

The *British Medical Journal* Clinical Evidence survey found that only 35 percent of 3000 medical practices were effective, 15 percent were damaging, and 50 percent of unknown usefulness. Other sources roughly agree, including Vinay Prasad (academic oncologist/epidemiologist at UCSF), the Robert Woods Johnson Foundation, and the Institute of Medicine.

The Congressional Budget Office estimates 30 percent of medical care is unnecessary. Other authorities using the "Milliman Health Waste Calculator" say useless therapeutic activities are 48 percent. John Ioannidis, MD, the Stanford statistician, asks, "How many contemporary medical practices are worse than doing nothing or doing less?" and concludes there has been a "decade of reversal" in therapies.

————

I ONCE THOUGHT the system put patients first. But I learned the brutal reality—almost everyone puts money first. The medical companies saw our blend of capitalism, insurance, and financial supports for the needy and moved in.

These corporations routinely buy their way out of colossal criminal accusations by paying fines up to hundreds of millions or even billions of dollars. A lot of what they do would be illegal or unethical for people, but it is within the letter of the law for corporations.

The following chapters tell the mind-bending tale of doctors, hospitals, and pharmaceutical and device companies heedlessly chasing trillions of dollars. It happened in an industry led by doctors, considered by many the best-trained, most ethical, and most intellectual group in America.

CHAPTER 4

INDUSTRY SEDUCES DOCTORS

Physicians, medical schools, and professional organizations have no… excuse, since their only fiduciary responsibility is to patients. [Their] mission… is not to enter into lucrative commercial alliances with the pharmaceutical industry. As reprehensible as many industry practices are, I believe the behavior of much of the medical profession is even more culpable.

— MARCIA ANGELL, FORMER EDITOR-IN-CHIEF, NEW ENGLAND JOURNAL OF MEDICINE (NEJM).

HOW COULD physicians have allowed this to happen? No doctor I know started with the idea of money above patients. We all wrote that essay in school about how we wanted to save the world. But we are now pawns of moneyed interests, and we often betray our patients' trust.

Physician training is brutal, and our expectations are high. Most of us have little income through our mid-30s, and we often take out huge loans. We may be responsible for spouses and children. Everyone around us seems to be squeezing a fortune out of healthcare: older surgeons, radiologists, hospital administrators, and even the lawyers suing us. We want to claw our way up the pay scale.

The best marketers on the planet are spending billions of dollars trying to get us to channel whatever resources we control towards their companies. We know this, yet we still connect with our patients, inspire their trust, and try to do our best. They are dependent on us, especially the sick ones, and this makes us responsible for all consequences.

I am by turns reverential and contemptuous of my peers. Some are true *mensches*. This Yiddish word means they are honorable, modest, and outstanding mentors. These real physicians are with us still, and you will hear their angry and sorrowful voices here. Others sacrifice their patients' health to make more money.

Most of us are somewhere in between. We are trying to make a living in a system where the industry has rendered the science murky. Most of our misdeeds are not intentional, and few of us admit to ourselves that we ever take advantage of patients. We are blind to our faults, but to the patient on the receiving end, it is a moot point.

Doctors imagine their scientific training and professionalism allow them to walk through this jungle without bias. But we are profoundly vulnerable, the more so because we believe little can sway us. Nothing excuses us for ignoring patients' best interests—not fatigue, confusion, ignorance, or even cowardice.

Salespeople begin our seduction in medical school, where they supply free food. Gangs of them later invade our offices. The corporations teach them the "three Fs of sales:" food, flattery, and friendship. Relationships are everything; the sales reps occasionally even use the fourth F. The target rarely understands what is going on, and the profits from blowing up prescribing are enormously larger than corporate marketing expenses.

Gifting has a considerable effect. Accepting a single pharmaceutical industry-sponsored meal produced higher rates of
prescribing. The more expensive meals had bigger effects.
Doctors who accept money prescribe brand-name medications twice as often. Recipients of industry funds write more
costly prescriptions. A JAMA review (2000) entitled "Is A Gift
Ever Just a Gift?" looked at 538 studies about lectures and
gratuities sponsored by drug companies. Gifts transformed
physician behavior. How could it not?

An analysis at Worstpills.org, published by the Ralph
Nader group Public Citizen, concluded that this situation
produces staggering overprescribing. In 2018, US patients
filled 4.19 billion prescriptions, *over 13 per person*. Since many
of us take no medications, the rest are consuming a freakish
quantity.

**How can presents have such a profound effect on profes-
sionals?** The answer lies in "influence theory," a foundational
field of psychology that corporate marketers have
weaponized to boost sales. Any time we give a gift or favor,
substantial leverage occurs. This is "reciprocity." It seems
obvious, but we are easily fooled.

People who help you have the favor returned. Turning
down gifts is antisocial, and we think of those who do not
give back as "moochers." Larger presents make a bigger
difference, but small ones can be powerful as well.

Reciprocity is likely a fundamental evolutionary survival
trait. Giving and receiving meals with strangers locks in relationships. In the past, this allowed a tribe or person to
support others during hard times when starvation loomed.
Food, from sandwiches for office staff to lavish dinners for
doctors, is one of the most potent weapons in the corporate
drive to increase drug and device sales.

Outside medicine, business people recognize reciprocity.
They scramble to gain an advantage by delivering favors,

even as small a consideration as holding a door. The impulse to return gifts is reflexive and powerful. This is unlike negotiated exchanges.

Restaurants that give free samples of food can make purchases seem irresistible. Drug companies provide samples of expensive drugs to doctors who then gift them to patients. The process bonds everyone to eventual purchase—which is often painless because insurance pays.

At one time, Hare Krishna's followers were handing out flowers at many US airports. This worthless gift often triggered an automatic contribution. The beggars would pocket the money, and the travelers would throw the flowers away. The Krishnas would then pick them out of the wastebaskets and reuse them. Another example: restaurant tips significantly increase when the waiter leaves candy with the check.

After reading about influence studies, I understood why drug companies give away all that plastic junk. Besides reminding us of brand names, free pens and coffee cups start reciprocal relationships. Later, dinners, trips, and even substantial research grants may be available. A few prescriptions of stratospherically priced drugs will pay for nearly anything. Congress recognized how potent this is and banned large presents for physicians—yet loopholes still abound.

Industry representatives overwhelm busy doctors with these influence techniques. Reciprocity or returning favors is only one type. Others include:

✪ Authority (if the physician leaders do it, it must be right)

✪ Liking and identification (what a nice drug rep, he plays golf just like me)

✪ Social proof (my competitors are doing it)

✪ Scarcity (the product is nearly gone, buy or prescribe it now)

The best reference for this process is Dr. Robert Cialdini's

Influence (1984). This book has been regarded as a bible of sales by generations of business people.

We idolize celebrities, giving them credit for almost anything, even sound judgment. The companies flood TV, movies, and the Internet with their endorsements. These combine authority, liking, and social proof. For example, Bob Dole helped create a new category of disease, erectile dysfunction. In 2002 Kathleen Turner discussed rheumatoid arthritis on Good Morning America and directed listeners to a website. She did not disclose that she was working for Wyeth, the manufacturer of the rheumatoid drug Enbrel. Cases like this have been in the news for over a decade.

Ninety-four percent of US physicians accept drug and medical device companies' gifts. Most of us only receive a few dollars a year for an occasional sponsored lunch at medical meetings. But twelve percent of US physicians get paid for research—or sham research—and the money is substantial. According to *ProPublica*, the total industry gifts to physicians were over $2 billion a year in 2018, including gifts, meals, speaking, travel, and consulting. They did not count research grants, but *openpaymentsdata.cms.gov* did. This website said the total was $9.35 billion for 2018 alone. You can look up how much each doctor received on either website.

There is now one pharmaceutical sales representative for every five doctors in the US. They call the big prescribers who like and use their drugs "whales." Companies often pay them to lecture about products at meetings. Hawking physician credibility like this has built many a summer home.

Jerome Kassirer, former editor of the NEJM, described all the payoffs in *On the Take* (2004). Some consultant physicians get free trips to Florida, some get $1000 for attending one-day meetings, and some get paid for allowing their names on ghostwritten articles.

Psychiatrists receive more money from corporations than

any other US specialty. Many hide the payments. Lisa Cosgrove studied the highly influential psychiatric diagnostic "bible," the *Diagnostic and Statistical Manual of Mental Disorders (DSM IV and V)*. She reported that three-quarters of the authors had financial ties to corporations.

Pharmaceutical companies know which of us is prescribing each medication. Here is how they find out. Although pharmacies will usually refuse to sell the names of doctors who prescribe, they will sell their Drug Enforcement Agency (DEA) numbers. The American Medical Association (AMA) then sells the doctor's name that matches each number back to the corporations. The companies find out precisely how much medication each physician prescribes. This allows them to pressure doctors to sell more and target those who are small prescribers or who do not use their products at all. Including this, the AMA made more than $56 million from database sales in 2018.

I know a family physician who gets a free dinner nearly every week. He recently had his housewarming party catered by a drug company. Specialists usually control more sales, and they often get the most. Everyone thinks this is harmless, but it is not.

Other industries criminalize this kind of behavior. For example, the Securities and Exchange Commission has clear rules about disclosure when raising money for investments. An investor needs to know conflicts that could effect returns, just as a patient should know if a corporation has paid the doctor to prescribe. Law, business, and governmental groups forbid outside relationships that produce financial gain, professional advancement, or family advantage. Ethical conflicts like these may provoke a lawsuit or criminal prosecution.

Lawyers can be disbarred for concealing conflicts of interest (COIs). Judges recuse themselves or are recused by their supervisors from involvement where they have personal or monetary relationships. Federal judicial and executive branch bureaucrats must sell their ownership in companies of industries that they might affect. The federal government prohibits its employees from accepting anything with a value of over $20. Reporters "may not take any payment, gift, service, or benefit... offered by a news source...[in order to] maintain accuracy, balance, and the truth."

Physicians' organizations are also being bought. The medical industry gives them trinkets, research grants, outright grants (sometimes in the millions), speaker's fees, and substantial exhibitor fees for their meetings. Free ghost-writing is part of it. All this ensures favorable guidelines, prescribing, and publications. One reviewer called the conferences "unprofessional conduct" and wrote that the impact of the system was overwhelming.

Nearly all the societies' websites state that they are "funded by an unrestricted grant from company X." Each physician group has policy statements saying they have no commercial bias, however. Their physician leaders vehemently proclaim objectivity with editorials in the journals.

For example, the Endocrine Society says in its Code of Ethics: "The Society actively seeks outside financial or in-kind support... from pharmaceutical, device, or biotech companies... [and they] maintain complete independence between industry support of any and all of its programs... [and] objectivity and credibility are not compromised in any way." However, for their "Endo2015" national meeting, they advertised the industry perks, from "therapy dogs" to raffles, to prizes, to local jazz artists. Posters on their website proudly stated (caps in the original):

WITH MORE THAN 5800 ATTENDEES, ENDO DELIVERED ON IT'S PROMISE TO PUT YOUR COMPANY AND BRAND IN FRONT OF THE LEADERS IN ENDOCRINE PRACTICE

They have over a dozen corporate sponsors. Implausibly, their "Statement on Industry Relationships," reminds us: "Sources of commercial support do not influence the scientific, educational or public policy decisions of the Society."

Companies now spend at least twenty percent of their vast marketing budgets on the physicians who have the most influence. They call them the "key opinion leaders," using the acronym KOL. Since routine gifts to physicians have been progressively restricted by federal law, the companies focus on things like study funding, which has few rules. This research money is used to induce top doctors to corrupt science, produce favorable conclusions, and advocate for products.

Many of these physicians conceal the sources of their money. For example, the dean of Yale's medical school, the director of a cancer center in Texas, and the incoming president of the most prominent society of cancer doctors all published articles in medical journals without disclosing financial ties to pharmaceutical and healthcare companies (*New York Times*, 2018). José Baselga, MD, chief medical officer at Sloan Kettering Cancer Center, took millions from industry, published frequently, but mostly kept the payments secret. When this came out, he resigned (*NYT/ProPublica*, 2018).

Industry pays the KOLs to write favorable guidelines for physician practice. Hundreds of these statements now command doctors to perform in ways that jack up drug sales. Four of five authors of these "standards" have financial relationships with the corporations, with an average of ten conflicts of interest (COIs) per contributor. One study looked at 431 guidelines. Eighty-eight percent had no disclaimers and did not even reference the relevant literature. A *JAMA* review of 279 guidelines produced by 69 authors concluded their methodological quality was atrocious. Unfortunately, these "standards of care" have the weight of expert testimony in court.

Gilbert Welch told how the corporations made it happen in *Overdiagnosed, Making People Sick in the Pursuit of Health* (2011):

> *The head of the diabetes cutoff panel [which established standards] was a paid consultant to Aventis Pharmaceuticals, Bristol-Myers Squibb, Eli Lilly, GlaxoSmithKline, Novartis, Merck, and Pfizer — all of which made diabetes drugs. Nine of the eleven authors of recent high blood pressure guidelines had some kind of financial ties... [to the medication manufacturers]. Similarly, eight of the nine experts who lowered the cholesterol cutoff were paid consultants of the drug companies making cholesterol drugs. And the first osteoporosis standard was established by... a panel... whose corporate advisory board consisted of thirty-one drug and medical equipment companies.*

The industry has even infiltrated medical schools, home to some of the most influential physicians. Eric G. Campbell, Ph.D., studied 459 department chairs of US medical schools. Two-thirds of them and two-thirds of their departments had close ties to industry. An overwhelming majority of these chief doctors believed they had no biases related to this.

In another study, he discovered that a third of the Institutional Review Board members who approve studies had corporate COIs. Thirty-five percent of them had conflicts regarding issues they voted on during the past year. Federal guidelines require recusal in these situations, but they are ignored.

Disclosure is used to launder conflicts of interest, but this gets nothing clean. Elsevier, the largest medical publication house, requires its authors to confess their payments in writing. But this does not disinfect payoffs. No matter how strong an argument, if it comes from a paid advocate, a balanced view is impossible. Sponsors punish actions contrary to their interests by cutting off their consultants' money.

Joseph Biederman, MD, has one disclosure statement of 364 words, an article in itself. He was censured for failing to disclose some of his many sources of corporate pay, and the *NY Times* asked whether he was an "expert or shill." He is Chief of Clinical and Research Programs in Pediatric Psychopharmacology and Adult ADHD at the prestigious Massachusetts General Hospital. Here is another disclosure statement:

> Dr. Gertz reports personal fees from Ionis/Akcea, personal fees from Alnylam, personal fees from Prothena, personal fees from Celgene, personal fees from Janssen, grants and personal fees from Spectrum, personal fees from Annexon, personal fees from Appellis, personal fees from Amgen, personal fees from Medscape, personal fees from Physicians Education Resource, personal fees for the Data Safety Monitoring board from Abbvie, personal fees from Research to Practice, speaker fees from Teva, speaker fees from Johnson and Johnson, speaker fees from Medscape, speaker fees from DAVA oncology, roles on the Advisory Board for Pharmacyclics and Advisory Board for Proclara outside the submitted work, royalties from Springer Publishing, and Grant Funding from Amyloidosis Foundation and International Waldenstrom Foundation; NCI SPORE

Everyone respects doctors, particularly those with fancy degrees and university affiliations. Credibility based on credentials seems dependable. Unfortunately, influence works on them the same as on the rank-and-file. After money changes hands, the recipient's recommendations about drugs, treatments, and surgery are biased. Pretensions of objectivity citing authority are much worse than nothing because they fool us. Patients and doctors alike are blind to this.

Neither physicians nor patients are tough-minded enough to believe that powerful effects—essentially bribery—now command nearly every move in healthcare. In theory, doctors and other caregivers put patients before finances, but corporations are designed as money-making machines. For them, patient outcomes are a distant consideration.

PART II
WELCOME TO DRUG WORLD

CHAPTER 5

BIG PHARMA PROLOGUE

*For ourselves, we shall not trouble you with specious pretenses…
and make a long speech that would not be believed… You know as
well as we do that right, as the world goes, is only in question
between equals in power, while the strong do what they can and the
weak suffer what they must.*

— *Thucydides, The History of the Peloponnesian
War*

THE US IS a nation of pill poppers. According to Bloomberg, nearly half of us take prescription drugs. The Mayo Clinic (2013) puts this figure even higher, a whopping 70%, with 20% of Americans taking five or more (verified by the Centers for Disease Control in 2019). This is absurd and obviously damaging, but doctors do not get it. How could this have happened, and who is responsible?

Abraham Katz, MD, summarizes this section: *The immensely wealthy and powerful pharmaceutical companies have become more and more entitled and emboldened over the past three decades. The FDA requires drug studies for patent approval, so "contract research groups" do trials that spoil science and make questionable medications look good. Mathematicians massage the numbers and bury data that do not support the drugs. Industry employees then write up the trials and send them to the FDA. Since more than half of the regulator's funding comes directly from corporations, approval is rarely an obstacle.*

After the FDA gives permission to sell the drug, corporate ghostwriters spin articles for publication. Then the companies pay prominent physicians to affix their names as authors, and medical journal editors with financial conflicts approve them. Since the journals are primarily funded by the drug industry, publication is nearly automatic. The prestigious authors and publications lend credibility to questionable drugs, devices, and physician practices.

While this happens, physician opinion leaders with transparent financial conflicts such as research grants create prescribing guidelines that minimize risks and exaggerate benefits. These standards of practice are poorly grounded in science, but they authoritatively command practicing doctors how and when to use drugs.

The subsequent marketing campaign goes directly to the public and to individual physicians. Few observers believe either is appropriate, but the former is worse. Along with this, another favored strategy is corporate-funded advocacy groups that disease-monger. This involves spinning horror stories that spread fear to sell drugs.

Dr. Katz is a pseudonym for a top physician who tutored me as I wrote this book. He dives into medical studies rather than backstroking through the summaries like the rest of us. I quote him to develop ideas and provide contrasting views.

CHAPTER 6

DRUGMAKERS GET AWAY
WITH ANYTHING

*It was a situation for despair, but there was no alternative but to
keep one's nerve.*

— Colonel Heinz-Gunther Guderian, a Panzer
commander facing the Allied invaders on D-day

Wendy Dolin learned the hard way about antidepressants.
Her husband Stewart threw himself in front of a train a week
after he started taking generic Paxil. Mr. Dolin's doctors gave
him the drug for job-related anxiety, but it creates intolerable
restlessness in three to five percent of people using it. He was
last seen pacing back and forth on the train platform.

He killed himself despite what his family thought was a
perfect life. His two grown children adored him, and he loved
his career, travel, skiing, and his work. He was happily
married to his high school sweetheart. When Ms. Dolin sued
the drug company, testimony established that it had hidden
Paxil-related suicides.

For two decades, while making billions of dollars, the
manufacturer had been quietly settling thousands of similar

cases. In 2017, Ms. Dolin won a three million dollar judgment. Her attorneys had spent a million dollars, but the company filed an appeal. It claimed that the original manufacturer was not responsible for subsequent generic versions of the medication.

The following story may be worse. David Carmichael took Paxil for two periods of several months each and felt suicidal each time. His doctor advised him that increasing his dose would decrease his stress. When he did, he went from suicidal to homicidal and killed his 11-year-old son. The circumstances indicted Paxil, and Mr. Carmichael believes it was the cause. Since blaming the drug was impractical for his legal defense, this was not brought forward at his trial. The court acquitted him of murder because he was believed to be temporarily psychotic, which means out of touch with reality.

SSRIstories.org has about 5000 first-hand news stories about situations like these. The drug companies claim that the drugs are bystanders and that the perpetrators are prone to violence. A half-hour spent on this website makes a compelling circumstantial case that the drugs are the cause.

Corporate criminals calculate they will make money even if they are caught, convicted, and fined.

The Ford Pinto's gas tank sometimes exploded when the car was rear-ended. Ford knew about it but risked more deaths and lawsuits. They calculated that this was cheaper than a recall. After about 500 people died in fires and hundreds of lawsuits were filed, the press discovered the coverup.

British Petroleum (BP) had criminally lax safety practices, so the Deepwater Horizon oil spill in the Gulf of Mexico was not a surprise to industry observers. Eleven people died, and the spill devastated the southern coast of Louisiana. By 2016, BP's settlements and restitution for manslaughter and other crimes were projected to exceed $62 billion. But since their annual gross revenues that year were $183 billion, this was just a cost of doing business.

Volkswagen AG faked their emissions testing. When this came out, it damaged their reputation, and their stock price dropped by a third. By 2016, the fines and settlements in the US alone were over $25 billion. Their gross revenue that year was $259 billion, so it was, again, just another cost of doing business.

Pharmaceutical corporations violate more criminal laws than any industry in *history*, as measured by their criminal settlements. The top 22 drugmaker payoffs since 2004 have their own *Wikipedia* page of shame. Nine of the ten largest companies are there, and five payments are for more than a billion dollars. The medical device companies' behavior is similar. Prosecutors allow these businesses to admit little and keep their executives out of jail if they pay up.

Besides psychiatric drugs, many other medications are killers. About 50,000 people die each year in the US from opioids, and until the recent street fentanyl crisis, two-thirds of these involved prescriptions. Hospital medication fatalities have been well known since a 1998 meta-analysis in JAMA. Out of 39 studies of millions of US patients, there were about 100,000 deaths in 1994 alone.

The renowned Danish physician and researcher Peter Gøtzsche estimated that the total annual drug-related fatalities in the US and Europe was 200,000. This included hospitals and outpatients. It is the third-highest cause of death after heart disease and cancer.

The primary way US federal prosecutors attempt to hold pharmaceutical corporations to account is for "off-label marketing." Physicians have flexibility for prescribing patient-by-patient, but corporations are only supposed to promote products for the reasons stated on the product information label. Nevertheless, drug representatives hound doctors to prescribe medicines in unsanctioned ways. They also pay experts to speak about these "off-label" treatments. Strangely, while promoting drugs for off-label use is illegal, hiring experts to promote the drugs off-label in the guise of continued medical education is lawful.

Examples of this brand of criminality follow.

✪ In 2012, GlaxoSmithKline (GSK) paid a record $3 billion settlement and agreed to plead guilty to federal criminal charges. It was then the single largest healthcare fraud settlement. The company was alleged to have marketed unapproved uses of medications, lied to physicians about safety, lied in medical journals, and illegally promoted drugs for children. This involved ten medications: Avandia, Wellbutrin, Paxil, Advair, Lamictal, Zofran, Imitrex, Lotronex, Flovent, and Valtrex. As usual, there were no admissions of wrongdoing. Their stock rose nearly two percent after the agreement made the news. GSK's gross receipts were $27 billion (2016), so the massive fine was a bit more than a single month's total revenue, another cost of doing business.

✪ In 2009, Pfizer accepted a $2.3 billion fine settling civil and criminal allegations for illegal marketing of their anti-inflammatory Bextra. John Kopchinski, a former Pfizer sales representative and whistleblower, said, "The whole culture of Pfizer is driven by sales, and if you didn't sell drugs illegally, you were not seen as a team player." It was the fourth Pfizer settlement within a decade and only sixteen days worth of their total revenue.

Eliot Spitzer sued GlaxoSmithKline when he was New York's attorney general. He said, "What we're learning is that money [fines] doesn't deter corporate malfeasance. The only thing that will work in my view is CEOs and officials being forced to resign and individual culpability being enforced (2004)." People need to go to jail.

Litigation records are the visible tip of an enormous iceberg of concealed graft. Even bribery of foreign government officials, as reflected in US criminal settlements, has become commonplace, as described in a 2017 *Public Citizen* article. The *BMJ* (formerly the *British Medical Journal*) describes scandals almost weekly.

Peter Rost, former Pfizer marketing vice president, compared the drugmakers to mobsters:

> *It's scary how many similarities there are between this industry and the mob... obscene amounts of money... killings and deaths... [bribing] politicians and others... The difference is, all these people in the drug industry look upon themselves... as law-abiding citizens... However, when they get together as a group and manage these corporations, something seems to happen... It's almost like when you have war atrocities; people do things they don't think they're capable of... because the group can validate what you're doing as okay.*

By 2002, the top 10 drugmakers' profits equaled those of all the other 490 Fortune 500 companies together. Drug manufacturers, showered with federal and insurance money, have 20-25 percent net profit margins. Pfizer's have been phenomenal:

51 percent in 2013
43 percent 2014
40 percent in 2017
44 percent 2018

Thriving industries which freely compete and are not state-supported average less than 10 percent net profit margins.

Courageous Cassandras introduced me to drug industry practices. Ben Goldacre, for example, wrote the following about drug studies:

> *Drugs are tested by people who manufacture them, in poorly designed trials, on hopelessly small numbers of weird,*

unrepresentative patients, and analyzed using techniques which
were flawed by design, in such a way that they exaggerate the
benefits of treatments... You can compare your drug with
something you know to be rubbish--a drug at an inadequate dose
perhaps, or a sugar pill... you could peek at your results halfway
through, and stop your trial early if they look good.

— *BAD PHARMA*, 2012

David Healy is an academic psychiatrist who wrote *Pharmageddon* (2012). He says that for twenty-five years the corporations have been fabricating diseases and syndromes and
then marketing the drugs to treat them. He also says that over
half of our pharmaceutical spending is for proprietary
medications with dubious benefits such as antidepressants or
statins. He calls the current drug approval system "research
misconduct on a grand, international scale."

**Ghostwriters paid by industry draft more than half of all
drug studies and even some textbooks.** Academics whose
careers depend on publication claim authorship and lend their
credibility. Editors at prestigious journals give these authors a
pass. At the same time that this misconduct is sanctioned,
students are crucified for plagiarism and medical licenses are
revoked for physicians who change patient records. These are
misdemeanors compared to the industry's murderous practices.

A *Guardian* article (2009) described how a pharmaceutical
company offered writing services to Dr. Healy to emphasize
"the main commercially important points" of an antidepressant. Their rewrite of his paper made a mediocre medicine
sound fantastic, so he took his name off the article. Healy
wrote that many drugs are about the same and that their sales
depend mainly on marketing.

When academic physicians want to author a paper, they
often approach a pharmaceutical company that has the

research, evaluation, and writing teams in place. Only ten percent of trials are still run inside the US because data scams are easier to pull off where there is less scrutiny. In *The Citizen Patient* (2013), Nortin Hadler adds:

> [Contract Research Organizations, CROs, are] contracted to test for efficacy rather than to try to disprove efficacy. The latter is sound science. The former is profitable. The CROs, the recruited physicians, and usually the patients all receive remuneration for their participation. Long gone are the days when drug trials were free of vested interests, conflicts of interest, marketing undercurrents, and fraud. Some scandals [involve] "paper patients" and data massaging.

Dr. Robert Fiddes, a Southern California family practitioner, developed a business doing medical studies with fabricated data. He said, "…most researchers are forced to cheat because drug companies issue requirements for test subjects that sound good in marketing material but are impossible to meet in the real world… anyone successful in the business was skirting the rules." He went to jail for 15 months after being convicted of research fraud.

Studies confirm that company money destroys study integrity. In a 2007 analysis of 192 studies of statin drugs, favorable outcomes occurred twenty times more often with drugmaker funding than with other sources of support. In a review of psychiatric medications, trials paid for by the companies were positive 78 percent of the time, while with outside funding, only 48 percent were favorable. In a survey of 161 studies about harmful chemical exposures, only 14 percent found adverse health effects when industry-funded, but 60 percent revealed harm when independently funded. Other reviews of hundreds of trials also confirm funding bias. Expert witness bias is a well-known analogous situation.

Lawyers, like corporations, pick witnesses who favor the viewpoint of whoever writes their check.

Forty percent of the studies of antidepressants remain unpublished, undoubtedly because they revealed that the drugs did not work. In the published trials, industry may remove data, ghostwriters may misrepresent the information, or they may switch patients into categories that change outcomes. Suicide, violence, and other issues may be under-reported or hidden. As the rules exist now, drug companies are entitled to conceal whatever study information they want because they own it. The administrators and patient-volun-teers sign gag contracts.

Another often-used hoax is to publish positive studies over and over. For example, a 2005 review from Cochrane, arguably the most respected source in medicine, found a Zyprexa research data set that showed up 142 times in various publications. Zyprexa's cost is many times that of older drugs, although it is not more beneficial.

John Braithwaite is a pharmaceutical company whistle blower and author of *Pharmaceuticals, Corporate Crime, and Public Health* (2014). He said that marketing departments dominate the drug companies. He described the concealed studies and the decline of innovation in favor of promoting established classes of medications that make quick profits.

He suggested applying whistleblower laws from the False Claims Act to corporate crime. Whistleblowers get a portion of settlements, which "privatizes law enforcement." These incentives work, but they are currently only used for fraud against the government. Braithwaite said corporate penalties should be criminal rather than civil. He believes "corporate capital punishment" is the only way to get their attention. This means government takeover and sale of all assets. He calls this "corporate execution."

Federal prosecutors are powerful, but unfortunately, we have given these companies such enormous resources that they can afford vast lobbying operations and rich political payments. This effectively squelches most laws that could hold them criminally accountable. The standards for criminal conviction are high, so these cases are also tough to prosecute against wealthy white-collar defendants. The prosecutors have discretion, and their culture is to leave the troublesome cases alone.

Civil suits have lower requirements for proof than criminal cases. Some plaintiffs' attorneys have made inroads against the corporations. As of the publication date of this book, Purdue Pharma and Insys, both guilty of premeditated mass-murder using opioids, are finally being bankrupted by plaintiffs' lawyers. Remarkably, another company purchased the Insys fentanyl spray out of bankruptcy, and they continue to sell it.

The pharmaceutical industry finances 50 to 70 percent of all physicians' continuing medical education (2015/2018). This was $1500 per doctor each year, or $700 million total. For research, in 1977, the industry was paying for 29 percent, but by 2009, it was 60 percent and by 2014, 86 percent. Very little of this was an issue 40 years ago, but now they even fund medical schools.

How did the drugmakers get so out of control? The pharmaceutical companies' 2019 gross revenue, the total amount spent on drugs worldwide, was over $1.3 trillion (1300 billion). This had increased from one trillion in 2014. It is more than the gross domestic product (GDP) of any country except the top fourteen.

This industry is more than twice the size of Big Tobacco, which has only $500 billion in yearly global revenue. The National Football League's gross receipts in 2018 were $14.5 billion. This would not have put it in the top ten pharmaceutical corporations, which had from $24 billion to $52 billion in revenues in 2019.

The drug industry claims its research budget justifies the

outrageous pricing. But they likely spend double this on marketing. Figures vary by company and source, but crudely, research is 14 percent, and marketing might be 20-25 percent of revenue. Marcia Angell, former editor of the *NEJM*, said marketing and administration together is 35 percent.

In 2003, a law slid through Congress stipulating that Medicare, the world's largest drug buyer, could no longer negotiate prices with corporations. The statute directed them to pay 106 percent of the companies' average wholesale price. Although this seemed reasonable, it allowed corporations to price-fix. The Veteran's Administration, which was not part of the deal, now pays only about fifty percent of the Medicare rate for each medication. Even the notoriously wasteful US military bargains with competing defense contractors.

The US pharmaceutical lobby paid to make this happen. They spent $4 billion from 1998 through 2018, more than aerospace, defense, and oil/gas combined. The finance sector had the only lobby that was close—$5.1 billion between 1998 and 2008, but this figure included campaign contributions.

The US is only 4.3 percent of the world population, but soon after this legislation passed, 75 percent of the drugmakers' worldwide profits and nearly half of all medication spending came from the US. The committee chairman who pushed the law through, Wilbert Joseph Tauzin II, retired to a $2 million a year pharmaceutical company job. A final, almost surreal detail is that half of these pharmaceutical companies are not based in the US and do not pay our taxes. *This law allowed these outsiders to gouge us right along with the domestic corporations.*

POSTSCRIPT: Several other government-fueled industrial sectors also have high profit margins. Sarah Chayes in *Thieves of State* (2015) says that, besides healthcare, these include energy and banking, with 20-25 percent profits. We support the wasteful defense industry, but it does not post numbers like these. Tobacco had direct subsidies until 2014 and still had about 14 percent net margins in 2019. These companies all receive "free" money from the government rather than having to complete for it in the marketplace. Chayes says this transforms them into criminal or near-criminal enterprises as measured by their prosecutions.

CHAPTER 7

"THE FDA PROTECTS THE BIG DRUG COMPANIES"

We don't have safe drugs. The drug industry more or less controls itself; our politicians have weakened the regulatory demands over the years, as they think more about money than patient safety; there are conflicts of interest at drug agencies; the system builds on trust although we know the industry lies to us; and when problems arise, the agencies use fake fixes although they know they won't work... If the American people knew some of the things that went on at the FDA, they'd never take anything but Bayer aspirin.

— Len Lutwalk, FDA scientist

The FDA, by spinelessly knuckling under to every whim of the drug companies, has thrown away its high reputation, and in so doing, forfeited our trust.

— Drummond Rennie, deputy editor of JAMA

IN RECENT DECADES, FDA oversight has broken down. An editorial in the *BMJ* (2015), "The FDA's New Clothes," said the vast majority of the drugs approved by the FDA from 1978 to 1989 were ineffective. One in five causes serious harm after approval. A second analysis by the same authors reports that 80 to 90 percent of the newest drugs were not improvements over older ones.

FDA whistleblowers have reported what was happening. Ronald Kavanagh, PhD, is a pharmacist who reviewed medications for the FDA from 1998 to 2008. Martha Rosenberg interviewed him:

> [The] honest employee fears the dishonest employee. There is also irrefutable evidence that managers at CDER (Center for Drug Evaluation and Research of the FDA) have placed the nation at risk by corrupting the evaluation of drugs and by interfering with our ability to ensure the safety and efficacy of drugs. While I was at FDA, drug reviewers were clearly told not to question drug companies and that our job was to approve drugs. We were prevented, except in rare instances, from presenting findings at advisory committees. In 2007, formal policies were instituted so that speaking in any way that could reflect poorly on the agency could result in termination. If we asked questions that could delay or prevent a drug's approval - which of course was our job as drug reviewers - management would reprimand us, reassign us, hold secret meetings about us, and worse. Obviously, in such an environment, people will self-censor…I frequently found companies submitting certain data to one place and other data to another place and safety information elsewhere so it could not all be pulled together and then coming in for a meeting to obtain an agreement and proposing that the safety issue is negligible and does not need further evaluation… Sometimes we were literally instructed to only read a 100-150 page summary and to accept drug company claims without examining the actual data, which on multiple occasions I found directly contradicted the summary document. Other times I was ordered not to review certain sections of the submission, but invariably that's where the safety issues would be. This could only occur if FDA management was told about issues in the submission before it had even been reviewed. In addition, management would overload us with huge amounts of material that could not possibly

*be read by a given deadline and would withhold assistance. When
you are able to dig in, if you found issues that would make you turn
down a drug, you could be pressured to reverse your decision or the
review would then be handed off to someone who would simply copy
and paste whatever claims the company made in the summary
document... One manager threatened my children - who had just
turned 4 and 7 years old - and in one large staff meeting, I was
referred to as a "saboteur." Based on other things that happened and
were said, I was afraid that I could be killed for talking to Congress
and criminal investigators... I found evidence of insider trading of
drug company stocks reflecting knowledge that likely only FDA
management would have known. I believe I also have
documentation of falsification of documents, fraud, perjury, and
widespread racketeering, including witnesses tampering and
witness retaliation.*

Of the 5,918 FDA scientists who responded to a 2006
survey by the Union of Concerned Scientists, a fifth said their
superiors asked them to exclude, alter, or falsely interpret
their conclusions. They were often pressured to approve
drugs despite safety concerns. A follow-up survey in 2011
found they feared retribution if they wrote about this in journals or spoke to the press. Many said that political and business interests affect the FDA's decisions. Over a third felt that
a superior had interfered with their work in the past year. The
Institute of Medicine reported the same year that there was
significant outside interference with the FDA's scientific
work.

———

EARLY HISTORY: The FDA's mission is to protect health by
evaluating and approving food, drugs, vaccines, tobacco,
supplements, cosmetics, blood transfusions, medical devices,
and veterinary products. The agency oversees 20 percent of

the US economy. The pharmaceutical companies are required to perform drug studies according to an elaborate set of rules and present them to the FDA.

The FDA made its reputation in the 1950s when it saved Americans from congenital disabilities caused by thalidomide. A German pharmaceutical company marketed this drug almost without prior study. Its use was for sleep, anxiety, and morning sickness of pregnancy. It was sold over-the-counter in West Germany and other countries.

In the rest of the world, at least ten thousand babies born from mothers who had taken the drug had missing limbs, eyes, and ears. Half the babies died. Many adults who took the drug had nerve damage.

A heroine FDA regulator had her doubts and stalled its approval. Thanks to her, the thalidomide tragedy here did not reach the scale that it did in Europe. But the company passed out unapproved thalidomide samples and performed two trials on 20,000 patients, resulting in patient harms. As a result, in 1962 the US passed laws that directed manufacturers to prove to the FDA their products worked and were safe before they market them. Prescriptions were required for new drugs.

In recent years, however, direct payments from drugmakers to the FDA took the oversight process hostage. Since 2002, pharmaceutical companies paid about two-thirds of the FDA's $4.7 billion budget through "user fees." This money from industry goes straight to the FDA, mostly during the patent process. Critics have said the companies should pay taxes instead. In 2007, four retired FDA commissioners agreed: the system creates the wrong incentives. Jessica Wapner, in a PLOS blog, wrote that the structure puts the FDA in the pockets of the drug industry.

Any student of influence understands how and why this works. The payments, totaling over $3 billion in 2016 alone, create enormous leverage. Michael A. Carome, Director,

Public Citizen's Health Research Group, concluded, "User fees fundamentally changed the relationship between the FDA and the pharmaceutical industry such that the agency now views the industry as a partner and a client, rather than a regulated entity." Megan McArdle coined a name for this in a *Bloomberg* article: *regulatory capture*. She says that the regulators who are in place "to tame the wild beasts of business instead become tools of the corporations they regulate."

Congress ignored naysayers and ratified the US arrangement again in 2017. The UK has similar issues. There, drug companies pay 70 percent of the budget of their corresponding regulatory agency, the National Institute for Health and Care Excellence (NICE). Worse: sizable and open industry payoffs occur *after* the approval process. These reward cooperative FDA advisors on the committees responsible for endorsing drugs.

In 2006, the FDA made it harder for a consumer to sue a pharmaceutical company for harm. The industry had been trying for decades to get such a law passed through the legislature. It finally influenced someone at the FDA to sneak the measure through as a simple regulation. This created immunity for manufacturers unless plaintiffs proved that a company intentionally committed fraud, which is a high legal barrier.

FDA safety officer David Graham said in a 2004 congressional hearing, "I would argue that the FDA, as currently configured, is incapable of protecting America against another Vioxx [a drug removed from the market for causing fatalities]... Simply put, the FDA and its Center for Drug Evaluation and Research are broken."

How it all started: In 1992, the FDA began a sped-up drug approval process. This was an incentive to get medicines to the market sooner in response to the HIV epidemic. They allowed "surrogate" outcomes such as lab tests rather than requiring "hard" clinical outcomes such as death or heart attack. And they mandated only a single study. The FDA approved the HIV drugs based on increases in the T white blood cell counts and decreases in blood virus counts. Post-marketing surveillance was to have accompanied the scheme, but the Agency never correctly implemented it.

After the start of the accelerated approval process, a review a few years later found that a full third of the drugs approved by the FDA had safety issues. But there were few recalls. They ultimately only took one medication in twenty off the market. If there was regulatory action, it usually consisted solely of a "black-box" warning on the drug label about the possibility of serious harm. The drugmakers bitterly opposed this step because it limits profiteering. For example, Singulair, a pricey asthma medication, causes psychiatric problems including suicide, but so far there is no black box because of industry resistance.

The FDA permits data scams. Researchers from the Yale University School of Medicine looked at trials between 2005 and 2012. They found that the FDA based many drug approvals on studies that used various forms of data cheating. Donald Light and Ben Goldacre separately confirmed this story. They wrote:

✪ Thirty-seven percent of the drugs had only a single study.

✪ Forty-five percent of the trials for drug approval used study endpoints such as blood sugar or cholesterol (surrogate markers) rather than hard endpoints such as death or another clinical finding.

✪ Nearly a third 0f all the studies made a comparison with an older drug. When two drugs are found to be about the same, the companies usually claim some obscure advantage for the recent one. This games the approval process and allows the industry to market expensive "me-too" medications that offer no benefit over the older ones.

✪ To make a drug look good, the companies often exclude

people who are more likely to have adverse outcomes. Other times, they use people who are more likely to have problems, which can make an older drug look bad.

✪ When companies do un-randomized trials on unrepresentative populations, they can create almost any result.

✪ Experiments are sometimes run that lack a comparator or control arm. This is called a single-arm trial and has little validity.

✪ Some experimenters do approval studies that are not randomized, controlled, and double blinded, which is the current standard of proof. Some allow studies that are easily unblinded.

✪ To show benefit, sometimes doses of a test drug are used that are too high for routine clinical use. These studies last long enough to show benefits but are kept short enough to conceal adverse reactions.

✪ The other way this is played is to use high doses of the comparison drug. This creates side effects that make the new drug look great by comparison.

✪ Another often-used ploy is inaccurate measurement and improper reporting of the number needed to treat and number needed to harm.

✪ Huge trials are sometimes stopped early because results appear beneficial or harmful at that point. This prevents full evaluation and complete reporting.

Physicians should be trained to detect these commonplace forms of deceit when reading medical journals. I spotted them as I learned more.

In a 2012 BMJ editorial analysis, Donald Light and Joel Lexchin wrote that, of all the new products developed in the past 50 years, 85-90 percent produced many harms but few benefits. Most of them are me-too drugs used for established markets. They are not improvements. These medications are 80 percent of the US increase in drug spending.

Despite the sad deterioration of the FDA, it is still the

most respected and active organization of its kind in the world. Many of its people are idealistic and well-meaning, and they try to maintain standards. They are the only barrier between US consumers and pharmaceutical disasters. To their credit, the FDA is mostly successful at keeping shoddy drugs out of the US. Foreign manufacturers sell these with impunity in Brazil, Africa, Mexico, and Eastern Europe.

POSTSCRIPT: The FDA lets the drugmakers create early expiration dates to ensure more sales. In a 2006 study of 122 expired drugs, two-thirds of them were stable in every tested lot. Their sell-by dates were over four years too early. The US military, the CDC, and the Department of Defense understand this and for decades have saved billions of dollars by stock-piling outdated drugs. But the Pharmaceutical Research and Manufacturers of America (PhRMA) lobby claims the short expiration dates are only about safety.

CHAPTER 8

DISEASE-MONGERING &
BOGUS CURES

I want to sell drugs to everyone. I want to sell drugs to healthy people. I want drugs to sell like chewing gum.

— Henry Gadsden (1976), former CEO of Merck,
which developed some of the first medications that
patients needed to take indefinitely, including the
statin Mevacor (lovastatin).

WE EXPECT hucksterism about the benefits of cars, clothes, and beauty treatments. But it surprises us when it comes from the medical industry, which uses identical marketing tricks. They frighten us with diseases to sell expensive drugs and treatments.

Here is how it works. Prominent physicians, guided by corporations, start with some ailment, real or imagined, and are paid to endorse therapies and drugs for it that are barely effective or sometimes even ineffective. But they do not stop there. They then promote more and more inclusive criteria for the "disease," which creates more patients who need to take more medications and have more treatments. Finally, charity groups funded and controlled by the companies promote public awareness campaigns targeting both doctors and patients.

More specifically, drugs are used to treat blood pressure, cholesterol, and diabetes to avoid stroke, heart attacks, diabetic blindness, and other diseases. To accomplish this, physicians are guided by numbers for blood sugar, blood pressure, and cholesterol. The numbers considered abnormal are being continuously exaggerated to expand the group that supposedly requires drugging. *This has made paying patients out of over half of us.*

For example, the diabetes definition was originally a fasting blood sugar of over 140 mg/dl. This was changed to 126, which instantly gave diabetes—and drugs—to tens of millions of Americans who previously thought themselves healthy. Abnormal cholesterol went from over 240 to anything over 200. This also supposedly requires medications. The blood pressure considered treatable was originally over 160 for the higher (systolic) number. Now, anyone over 130 may get a medication prescription. None of these changes was dictated by substantial science, and all made a massive amount of money.

This has been established industry strategy for decades. Vince Parry explained it in *Medical Marketing & Media* (2003). He gave this conspiracy gravitas by dubbing it "Condition Marketing:"

> *There are three principal strategies for fostering the creation of a condition and aligning it with a product:*
> - *elevating the importance of an existing condition*
> - *redefining a current condition to reduce a stigma*
> - *developing a new condition to build recognition for an unmet market need.*

The expense and anxiety of having a diagnosis are not the only problems for patients. Sometimes the wrong treatment is performed, and sometimes surgical complications occur. Prescription medications are a major source of errors and even deaths. The Institute of Medicine states that medication errors cause demise for one of 131 outpatient and 1 of 854 in-hospital deaths.

Lower blood pressure occasionally causes fainting, which is a disaster when driving. Drugs that lower blood sugar can cause blackouts or even death. Cholesterol medications create a host of problems, including occasional deaths because of muscle damage.

Drugs may be worth the risk of side effects for sick people whose disease process is being treated. However, people who take drugs unnecessarily enjoy none of the benefits. They still suffer side effects, which are the only effects for them. Anyone not stuck in the tar-pit of recent medical thought would think this was beyond obvious. Drugs, treatments, and lab tests must be reserved for the ill, *who have symptoms.* The following diseases show how far our current practices have departed from this simple, traditional standard.

Diabetics cannot absorb sugar (glucose) from the blood into the body properly. This causes high blood sugar levels that, over time, produce blindness, heart attacks, kidney failure, and even death. The discovery and use of insulin to facilitate glucose absorption and thus lower blood sugar levels are among medicine's finest achievements.

People with childhood or type 1 diabetes cannot get glucose out of the blood into the body because they make no insulin. They require daily injections to survive. People with type 2 diabetes, who are mostly older, still produce it, but their bodies are resistant to its effects. We treat them with diet and oral medications to decrease their blood levels, and some doctors give them insulin. The benefits of drugging this group are controversial, especially for insulin and especially in older patients.

The new, expensive oral medications for type 2 diabetes

are associated with increased heart attack deaths. Despite their high cost, patients taking them do not live longer than those on the older diabetic medications. This should have eliminated their use altogether.

Avandia was probably the worst offender in this class, yet by 2006 the drugmakers promoted it into becoming the highest-earning diabetic drug in the world. It lowers blood sugar, but as with the others, it increases heart attacks and deaths. Thirteen thousand lawsuits have been filed against the manufacturer, and they settled 11,500. Endocrinologists have been vocal in opposing it, and it is no longer available in Europe, but the drug is still sold in the US[1].

The profits from these medications defy imagination. Their worldwide revenues, including the insulins, were $27 billion in 2008 and $71 billion by 2015. This involves many companies. Dr. Gøtzsche reported (2013) that the manufacturers structured the studies of the newer oral blood sugar drugs to conceal fatalities. Rather than carefully testing patient outcomes, the trials looked at surrogate numbers such as sugar and hemoglobin A1c, which is a measure of glucose values during the three months before the test is performed.

Metformin was first used in 1922. It helps with weight loss, lowers blood sugar, and lowers hemoglobin A1c. It does not create hypoglycemia when used alone and likely decreases deaths and heart attacks. Lifestyle changes should always be tried first for type II diabetes, but if any drug is used, metformin is the cheapest and safest. The recently patented drugs are not an improvement.

Likewise, the purpose of blood pressure control is to prevent heart disease and stroke. The Cochrane Collaboration (2012) looked at the studies and saw no evidence that reducing blood pressures below 160/100 improved health. In 2018, they evaluated studies of patients with heart and vascular disease and found the same thing. For older adults, another review (2017) found no evidence that the lower numbers helped either.

The massive SPRINT study published in 2017 supported tighter blood pressure control. Although this was primarily a government-funded trial, detractors pointed out that the study design was flawed. They also used wrong blood pressure machines, and some calculations were in error.

The American College of Cardiology (ACC) at one time defined high blood pressure as higher than 160/100. They dropped this to 140/90, and then in 2017 to 120/80 for some patients. The American Heart Association has the nerve to disease-monger this latest guideline using photographs of men who have scars down the center of their chests after coronary artery bypass grafting. The ACC is threatening a monstrous surgery that seldom helps anyone if people cannot get their blood pressure down to a reading that makes no known difference! Our patients are now racing to the emergency room in fear of strokes if they see 160/100 on their home blood pressure machines.

Everyone seems to have forgotten that statin anti-cholesterol medications are another attempt to prevent heart attacks. But the FDA approved them solely because they changed numbers. The vast majority of patients using statins have no known heart disease and no other issues. These patients do not live any longer. A study published in PLOS (2016) looked at over a million person-years of data and concluded the drugs are prescribed for many who do not benefit, and that the prescribing guidelines are wrong. In women, they slightly reduce the risk of events such as heart attacks, but they do not improve longevity (1998). The JUPITER trial, published in 2009, confirmed this. This information is ignored.

If 83 men who have already had a heart attack or another cardiac event take the drugs for five years, one in 83 will have his life saved, but the medications cause muscle damage in

one in 10 and diabetes in one in 50. For the rare case of hereditary high cholesterol, defined as about twice normal, there are
also slight advantages. But for the vast majority, statins cause
more harm than good. At least 18 percent of users have a
recognized side effect. These include sexual dysfunction and
Parkinson's disease. One in 204 gets diabetes. Muscle damage
occurs in one in 21, and this is occasionally fatal.

Despite this, the industry wants us to use statins routinely
for healthy people. Their excuse is that the drugs prevent
heart attacks and strokes in a few—despite not affecting *lifespan*. Guidelines from the American College of Cardiology
and the American Heart Association (2013) recommend that
12.8 million Americans and a *billion people worldwide* take the
drugs. Over half of the committee members who invented
this idea had a financial connection with the pharmaceutical
industry.

The FDA approved the drugs for children with hereditary
high cholesterol, defined as about twice-normal for both total
and "bad" cholesterol. The studies have never shown a longer
life span for treated children. Yet the pediatric society recommends checking cholesterol three times during the years from
2 to 18, citing the obesity rates as justification.

TheNNT.com is a website devoted to summarizing which
treatments work and which do not. They promote a simple
way to understand statistics—calculating the number of
people that are needed to be treated to produce one beneficial
patient effect. They say the following about statins: "Virtually
all of the major statin studies were paid for and conducted by
their respective pharmaceutical company. A long history of
misrepresentation of data and occasionally fraudulent
reporting of data suggests that these results are often much
more optimistic than subsequent data produced by
researchers and parties that do not have a financial stake in
the results…"

John Abramson reviewed the situation in *The Pharmaceu-*

tical Journal in 2015. Like *theNNT.com*, this is for an academic audience. His sense of outrage percolates through his careful verbiage: "The bottom line is that practically all that we think we know about the efficacy and safety of statins has been brought to us by commercial interests that hold the actual data as proprietary secrets… we cannot verify commercial claims of efficacy and safety."

The purpose of osteoporosis treatment is to prevent fractures, which have a relationship to fatality. Half the women over 50 will get an osteoporotic fracture, and by the time Americans are 65 years old, 20 percent of all of us, 300,000 per year, will have broken our hips. For women, the studies of deaths happening within a year after this vary between 14 to 58 percent. The annual deaths from breast cancer are about 42,000, which is roughly similar.

Do these deaths related to hip fracture occur in already debilitated people, or do the breaks cause deaths or both? The answers are not clear, nor are the benefits of the therapies we use. But since fractures in the elderly are a major problem, prevention of some sort seems reasonable to nearly everyone.

The drugs promoted for the prevention of bone thinning are the bisphosphonates, but they are worse than nothing. They are expensive, ineffective, increase fracture rates, and even cause rotting jawbones for some people. TheNNT.com summarized the data, quoting a Cochrane meta-analysis. They report that the medications prevent fractures solely in the group of women who have both osteoporosis shown on a scan plus a previously broken bone.

The drug industry aggressively promoted biphosphonate drugs using the standard methods of disease-mongering and diagnosis-creep. It all began at a Rome medical meeting in 1992 when the doctors concocted the pre-osteoporosis state of "osteopenia." They defined this as decreased bone density found on a radiologic study, diagnosed using an invented threshold, and without symptoms. The manufacturer released

Fosamax, the first drug to treat it, at about the same time. Although you can find contrary information about the "controversies" on the Internet, there is no proof these drugs decrease clinically significant fractures.

Merck, the Fosamax manufacturer, began building thousands of machines to permit physicians to check bone density in the wrist or other areas of the arms or legs. However, although bone density in the spine or hip predicts fractures, these locations do not. Merck got the machines FDA-approved, funded leasing programs for physicians, and somehow the scans were soon reimbursed by Medicare. The drugmaker understood that when physicians made money doing scans, the entire scam would blast off. In further marketing ploys, Merck launched a nonprofit, the Bone Measurement Institute, along with a massive disease awareness campaign. Soon, nearly every woman had something more to worry about.

The entire thing seemed credible to the US Preventive Services Task Force (USPSTF). Their process is to select a handful of doctors and have them vote on an issue. Despite the dubious history, they put together a group who ratified the use of these drugs for osteopenia, this symptomless scan finding which has only a theoretical relationship to fracture.

Merck was still not content. They were soon able to liberalize the bone density numbers considered diagnostic for their invented disease. Medical standards (in this case medical mythology), now recommends these drugs for 52 percent of all senior women. Sales have soared, of course.

Tens of millions of women now use these risky biphosphonates. Fosamax alone sold about $3 billion in 2007 before it went off patent. This declined to $284 million by 2016, but other drugs replaced it. There are now ten of these medications with many manufacturers. Even though their popularity declined somewhat after their tendency to *cause* fractures

became well known, the cost is many billions of dollars a
year.

**Influenza is self-limited to a few weeks and rarely
causes fatality or long-term disability.** Treatment and
prevention are part of the latest trend to profitably medicate
less severe diseases.

The corporations and their paid supporters claim Tamiflu
decreases flu symptoms and prevents complications such as
pneumonia. But the best estimate of benefit is that it may save
a half-day of sickness per individual per dose when
prescribed immediately after the start of symptoms. This is
nearly impossible. The FDA's longstanding opinion is that
Tamiflu did not affect complications, hospital admissions, or
survival. It prohibited the manufacturer from making these
claims.

A 2014 Cochrane review concluded the drug was worthless. They included many studies not sponsored by industry.
Two meta-analyses said risks were higher than the benefits.
Within a day of getting the drug, panic attacks, delusions,
convulsions, and even suicide have been reported. Complete
information is scarce, however. Study data withheld by the
manufacturer would reveal the entire truth, but so far, there
have been no legal challenges to get it. Industry sources,
including John Bell (Professor of Medicine at Oxford),
stonewalled Cochrane's requests for access to Roche's unpublished Tamiflu studies. He was on the board of directors for
Roche, and they paid him €322,450 in 2011.

Well-referenced reviews in the Huff Post and the Atlantic
report that Tamiflu does not decrease the chances of pneumonia or other severe illnesses. They also describe the
obscene marketing—or rather mongering—by Hoffmann-La
Roche and the Centers for Disease Control (CDC). Despite all
this, the medication had $18 billion in sales (2017). The US,
Britain, and other countries were somehow cajoled into stock-
piling billions of dollars' worth.

The CDC itself is compromised by millions of dollars in pharmaceutical company donations. They claim, however: "Our planners and our content experts wish to disclose they have no financial interests or other relationships with the manufacturers of commercial products… [the] CDC does not accept commercial support."

The label *scamiflu* instead of Tamiflu went viral on the Internet. A UK National Health Service analysis (2014) agreed: "The modest benefits of Tamiflu… do not justify the increased adverse risks, let alone the money spent on them." The WHO belatedly removed Tamiflu from their essential medications list in 2017.

The flu vaccine, just like Tamiflu, supposedly prevents pneumonia and other serious problems for those who are old or sick. Cochrane had grave doubts about this, however. They reviewed 90 flu vaccination studies and considered less than 10 percent of them decent science. Industry primarily funded the trials. Cochrane said:

> *Inactivated vaccines can reduce the proportion of healthy adults (including pregnant women) who have influenza and influenza-like-illness, but their impact is modest. We are uncertain about the effects of inactivated vaccines on working days lost or severe complications of influenza during the flu season.*

Despite this, the Centers for Disease Control (CDC) recommends the vaccine for nearly everyone and the World Health Organization (WHO) recommends it for vulnerable groups. Many hospitals shame nurses who refuse to get vaccinated into wearing surgical face masks, and a few even get fired. This is a $4 billion industry worldwide, and $1.6 billion is spent in the US.

Xigris was a drug for sepsis, which is an overwhelming infection that most often affects people at death's door. A split vote of an FDA advisory committee approved the drug after a single study purported that it worked. Eli Lilly was hoping for a billion-dollar blockbuster, and in 2001, they claimed the drug was "one of our industry's genuine breakthroughs." Their charges were $8,000 per patient.

The company hired a PR firm, who recommended they boost demand by claiming that Xigris was in short supply and needed rationing. This is the scarcity marketing ploy: buy it now; it is nearly gone. Eli Lilly's public relations firm started Surviving Sepsis, a nonprofit group supposedly representing patient interests. Lilly funded a campaign with the same name. Doctors with financial ties to Lilly created guidelines for the medication's use. Despite all this disease-mongering, they withdrew the drug in October 2011 because it was ineffective. Cochrane reported (2012): "All trials had high risk of bias and were sponsored by the pharmaceutical industry (Eli Lilly). We found no evidence suggesting that [Xigris] reduced the risk of death in adults or children with severe sepsis or septic shock. On the contrary, [it] increased the risk of serious bleeding."

Strokes occur when blood clots, cholesterol, or bleeding block parts of the brain's circulation. This causes brain dysfunction and sometimes partial or complete brain death.

"Clot-dissolving" medications (intravenous thrombolytics/tissue plasminogen activator/TPA) are FDA-approved for heart attacks. They occasionally help if given early. However, the emergency treatment of a stroke with these agents is questionable. A 2013 review showed no improved survival and some patient harm. Despite this, the FDA approved stroke treatment with these drugs.

Cochrane's 2009 report of 26 studies said the drugs produced, "an increase both in deaths (evident at seven to ten days and at final follow up) and in symptomatic intracranial haemorrhages." But in 2014, Cochrane reversed their opinion and said thrombolytic therapy was valuable if given in the first six hours. Since they had added only one inconclusive study to the primary analysis, this conclusion outraged knowledgeable commentators, who speculated that industry financing had infiltrated Cochrane.

These medications cost tens of thousands of dollars per patient wholesale. The hospital retails them for astronomically more. If knowledgeable physicians refuse to give them, hospital administrators may ask less ethical doctors to write the order. I interviewed Jake, the chief emergency physician for a group that believed intravenous thrombolytics do not work for stroke. His team told the hospital administrators they would not use them. So the hospital hired neurologists to Skype the emergency nurses and order the medicine hooked up. It costs $25,000 per patient just for the drugs, and the neurologists get paid just for phoning it in.

Jason is a radiology technician at another Los Angeles hospital. He told me the same story about the same specialists in his hospital's emergency department.

Prostate cancer treatment with Lupron is one of urology's embarrassments. This is a "chemical castration" medicine, approved in 1985 to treat metastatic prostate cancer. It did not sell well until the company figured out a way to pay off the surgeons. They developed a long-acting monthly shot, and urologists could buy it wholesale and retail it in their offices. This was a nasty conflict of interest that makes patient care secondary.

The company increased the temptation further by giving the doctors samples. This enticed them to sell the freebies to patients and keep the money, which is illegal. Medicare paid $1200 for one of these shots. Urologists could make several hundred thousand dollars a year on this. Internally, the manufacturer called these doctors their "drug whores." Lupron treatments accounted for 40 percent of all Medicare payments to some of these practices in the late 1990s.

After a whistleblower lawsuit and years of litigation, federal prosecutors settled this "nationwide conspiracy" with the manufacturer for $885 million. No corporate executives went to prison. The industry now skirts illegality by paying doctors an administration fee for using Lupron instead of providing free samples.

The worst part of this story is that Lupron is an atrocious drug. Men feel terrible, get hot flashes, and become impotent. Some have weight gain, fatigue, muscle loss, anemia, Alzheimer's disease, and osteoporosis. It also causes strokes, heart attacks, diabetes, and sudden death.

Otis Brawley, former head of the American Cancer Society, says men are dying earlier because of Lupron therapy. This drug and others have decreased prostate cancer deaths by 30 percent since 1990, but all-cause deaths have increased because the drug is so toxic:

> Widespread use of [anti-] hormonal agents is causing men to die of cardiovascular disease and diabetes before they would ordinarily die of prostate cancer. That's what I suspect is taking place. If urologists stop prescribing these drugs as widely as they used to, we will see deaths from prostate cancer inch up. That could be good news. Some men who would have died earlier with strokes and heart attacks caused by hormonal treatments of their asymptomatic disease would now live long enough to die of their prostate cancer.
>
> — HOW WE DO HARM (2012)

My friend Paul had his PSA checked every year. When he was 73, it jumped up to 10. Even though Paul felt fine, he went off to see the urologists, who obligingly biopsied his prostate. They found a tumor and now block his testosterone with a Lupron shot every few months. Medicare pays them a nice injection fee. Paul feels terrible because his testosterone levels are low.

Estrogen is likely a far better treatment. It is cheap; it works for many, and it has few side effects. Fifty years of experience shows it controls metastatic prostate cancer and does not feminize men. Since the companies cannot patent substances identical to those in the human body, they do not promote drugs like this. (Occasionally, delivery systems such as the estrogen patch or a supposedly unique drug strength is used to justify patent protection. For these medications, windfall profits can still be made.)

I'm not sure where drug marketers can go next. They already claim that nearly half of us have pre-diabetes, and forty percent of us have high cholesterol. One in six US citizens has already started on psychiatric drugs, for the claim is that half of us or more will have mental diseases during our lifetimes. The next few chapters show how they bully consumers and competitors and pull other dirty tricks to make more money.

CHAPTER 9

PHARMA'S MARKETING AND BULLYING

One of the benefits, if you are Pfizer, with illegal marketing is that the bell, once rung, cannot be un-rung. Doctors and patients remember the illegal messages, like that of Neurontin treating bipolar disorder, even if they are disavowed and found false. So despite the fact that Neurontin is approved only for epilepsy and postherpetic neuralgia [pain after shingles] it made Pfizer $387 million in 2008, and over 90 percent of sales were for its illegally marketed off-label uses.

— MARTHA ROSENBERG, BORN WITH A JUNK FOOD
DEFICIENCY (2015)

INTRODUCTION BY DR. KATZ: *We overpay the big pharmaceutical corporations for their drugs with tax and insurance funds, and then they use the money to carpet-bomb the Internet and media with marketing. They hijack legitimate advocacy groups and charities into this process with massive donations. They create some of these organizations out of whole cloth to promote sales.*

Direct-to-consumer ads blanket the media. These are illegal almost everywhere else in the world. The corporations promote virtually any drug that sells. There is little regard for the side effects of medications or the patient anxiety when they are labeled with a diagnosis. We now use medications without legitimate medical use for a vast swath of the population. I believe we should use drugs solely for sick people, where they have some chance of having more utility than toxicity. Even for these patients, we must do our best to not let our attempts to help cause harm.

Corporate marketing rules the Internet. Forests of junk ads and ghost-written articles are used to tout diseases and expensive remedies. Legitimate websites sell links, which the companies use for advertising. The ubiquitous corporate presence gets rewritten and shifts daily. It encourages the consumption of any profitable therapy.

The WebMD health network operates multiple websites including *WebMD.com, Medscape* (a well-liked medical news site), *MedicineNet, eMedicine, eMedicineHealth, RxList, Theheart.org,* and *Medscape Education.* This group collectively has revenues of $705 million a year (2016) and dominates medical information sources. According to Senator Chuck Grassley's investigations, the WebMD consortium is "shilling for the pharmaceutical companies and is a source of 'pseudomedicine and misinformation.'"

Here are the first words of one of the *WebMD* pages: "If you have bipolar disorder, the right medications can be like a pair of eyeglasses. Bipolar distorts your view of yourself and the world, but the medicine can help you to see things clearly again." A talented copywriter must have written this. But these medicines are of limited utility and are phenomenally overused. There is no objective test for bipolar disorder, no way to rule it out, no physical cause has ever been identified, and the drugs are uniformly harmful to health.

Epocrates.com is a favored application for physicians to look up drugs and patient-care information. Two Stanford students founded it in 1998. According to the website, half of US physicians and a million members use it.

Epocrates bombards users with specifically targeted ads.

The drugmakers supplied at least 70 percent of their $104 million revenue (2010), and the top 20 drug companies all buy ads. A former CEO, Kirk Loevner, described its profitability in a 2009 interview. He said *Epocrates* was a "gold mine" because of industry spending. They list the BioTech industry, including pharmaceutical and device companies as business partners on their website. People with ties to corporations manage the site. For example, Rosemary Crane, a former executive for both Bristol Meyers Squibb and Johnson and Johnson, was CEO for a period. Despite all this, the site's reputation is still excellent[1].

Drug companies now supply the lion's share of the patient advocacy groups' money. These were mostly created in good faith by idealists, and we still hold them in high regard. They exist for nearly every malady, from heart disease to Alzheimer's to mental health. People who have the disease and their family members often staff them, and many work for little or no pay. Consumers trust their websites.

But now, industry dominates agendas because the advocacy people have accepted funds. They additionally get expert guidance and political influence, but the price is giving up their control. The corporations expand "awareness" programs. They lobby Congress for early approval of "cures." They improve corporate images, and they sell drugs. It seems like a bargain to the nonprofit leaders.

The industry builds some of these societies from scratch, which is known as "astroturfing." These look like grassroots groups, but corporations fund, rent offices, and dictate agendas for them. They claim to represent the public but are corporate propaganda machines. In the US and many other countries, some of these practices are illegal, and the Federal Trade Commission has the power to impose hefty fines. Enforcement is difficult, however.

Jeanne Lenzer in *The Danger Within Us* (2017) described

how the companies maneuver advocacy groups and manipulate patients into giving testimonials before Congress:

It's a well-worn path of high farce: industry effectively launders its money through third-party organizations, and everyone acts as if it isn't happening. The process is akin to Congress inviting only the winners of million-dollar lotteries to testify about the "benefits" of gambling. Losers are not invited. Selection is everything, and as the saying goes, "Dead men tell no tales." What is not reported is equally as important as what is reported.

Although well-established medications have risks, poorly tested new ones are mostly complete failures. When adequate studies are never performed, the facts are never discovered. Few physicians and even fewer patients understand how difficult it is to prove a drug is worthwhile. The following groups advance industry agendas:

Eli Lilly, the Zyprexa manufacturer, bankrolled phony consumer groups that blasted the Kentucky state capital when the Medicaid program attempted to dump their expensive drug. There were emails, letters, hearings, and demonstrations. Lilly funded the whole uproar.

Citizens for Better Medicare started in 1999, yet somehow raised and spent $65 million fighting drug regulation in the 1999-2000 election. Tim Ryan, formerly the advertising director for PhRMA, the drugmakers' lobbying organization, was the executive director. He supported industry issues with millions of dollars in advertising. This society seems to have vanished from the Internet as of 2020.

Seniors Coalition and The United Seniors Association supported the disastrous 2003 law prohibiting the federal government from negotiating Medicare drug prices with industry. Public relations firms, which also represented the major drug companies, funded these groups. Neither had an office address or a membership list.

Ciba/Novartis, the manufacturer of Ritalin, gave Children With Attention Deficit Disorder (CHADD), a nonprofit, $1 million. This was a secret until a PBS documentary made it public. A daft Ciba representative said that CHADD was "essentially a conduit" for Ciba and Ritalin. In 2015, the industry supplied 27 percent of the organization's total revenue of $2.6 million. CHADD was responsible for most of the lobbying to include ADHD as a disability under the Individuals with Disabilities Education Act.

The National Alliance on Mental Illness (NAMI) claims on its website to be "the nation's largest grassroots mental health organization dedicated to building better lives for the millions of Americans affected by mental illness." They say they have over a thousand chapters in the USA. US Senator Chuck Grassley investigated them for not disclosing their pharmaceutical company funding. He forced them to release documents confirming that the industry provided a majority of their revenues. They now list their corporate donors on their website, including Lilly, GSK, AbbVie, Allergan, PhRMA (the pharmaceutical companies' lobbying organization), and Hospital Corporation of America Foundation.

Their focus is to encourage psychiatric medication use. NAMI's website says, "Even though most people can be successfully treated, less than half of the adults in the US who need services and treatment get the help they need." They allegedly coordinate their efforts with the drug companies to promote industry-favorable legislation[2].

Alzheimer's Society of the UK has over 2,500 employees, 10,500 volunteers, and annual revenues of £97.9 million. There is a similar but smaller group in Canada. The families of demented patients do not have this kind of money to donate. This group receives revenue from multiple drug companies and passes out about $100 million a year in research funding.

The UK Alzheimer's Society pushed a program that paid doctors a commission for each patient that they identified with Alzheimer's disease. This is an irresistible incentive. It frightened many people needlessly into believing they were becoming senile and promoted ineffective, phenomenally costly medications. In 2008, JR Gilstad and collaborators reviewed Aricept, one of the Alzheimer's medications, and found that if it had any benefit, it was modest. But the Alzheimer's Society's ads proclaimed, "Don't wait, ask your doctor about Aricept." When they tried this tactic in the US, the FDA informed them it was illegal.

The manufacturers of the sleep drugs Sonata and Ambien, plus the maker of the opioid OxyContin, together fund much of the National Sleep Foundation's budget. This nonprofit has sold a lot of addictive medications.

Alliance for Patient Access is an opioid lobby associated with over two dozen pharmaceutical companies, including Pfizer and Purdue Pharma. Their narrative is that legitimate pain patients should not pay the price for the fight against drug abuse.

The fake charities used to donate copays for phenomenally overpriced drugs are even worse. This seems like a generous idea, but it allows corporations to harvest massive insurance payments and gouge insurance almost without limit.

Here is how it works. If the physicians waive the co-pays, it is a fraud, because it violates the insurance contract. The drug companies cannot pay this money directly because it would be bribery. Medicare patients cannot legally accept a donation from a foundation owned by a pharmaceutical company. These "charities" skirt the Medicare anti-kickback laws by *concealing the donors' identities*. The last vestige of common sense—the patient's displeasure with drug costs—vanishes.

These "patient assistance foundations" give away $700 million a year to fund drugs that often cost more than $5000 a year per prescription. "Charities" like these cost the manufacturer nothing because the increase in sales is so much more than the money donated for a "copay assistance program." Later, after the insurance companies who are footing the bill have to raise their rates, we all pay. AbbVie and Johnson and Johnson are among the companies that play this game.

Direct-to-consumer (DTC) ads brainwash patients to pressure their doctors for brand names. Physicians usually obey rather than wasting time arguing, but almost everyone understands that these ads are a malignancy. Jerry Avorn, MD, wrote in the *NY Times*: "[This] advertising promotes only the most expensive products, it drives prescription costs up and also encourages the 'medicalization' of American life: the sense that pills are needed for most everyday problems that people notice, and many that they don't." Other experts agree.

The early 1980s, before the DTC ad strategy developed, were a more innocent and idealistic era. The following industry executives said that these ads hurt patients (1982).

Direct-to-consumer] advertising would make [patients] extraordinarily susceptible to product promises.

— CHARLES HAGAN, VP, AMERICAN HOME PRODUCTS

We believe direct advertising to the consumer introduces a very real possibility of causing harm to patients who may respond to advertisements by pressuring physicians to prescribe medications that may not be required.

— ABBOTT LABORATORIES CHAIRMAN

Advertising would have the objective of driving patients into doctors' offices seeking prescriptions.

— CHARLES COLLINS OF SMITH KLINE AND FRENCH

In the mid-1980s, a Madison Avenue advertising agency hired by Merrell Dow marketed Seldane, a new antihistamine. The FDA required ads to contain comprehensive warnings about side effects. The ad agency got around this by not explicitly naming the drug. They said, "ask your doctor," about how to treat allergies without sleepiness, which was drug's selling point. The campaign's enormous success spawned imitators. Then, by the late 1990s, court decisions allowed ads that had only a brief mention of side effects.

In 2001, the industry spent $2.4 billion on DTC ads, by 2008, $4 billion, and by 2016, $5.6 billion. These ads are now dramatic, frightening, and ubiquitous. These ads are only a portion of the drugmakers' marketing budget. By 2016, $5.5 billion a year was also being thrown directly at doctors to promote drugs. This is more than the yearly budget for educating all US medical school students.

Only the US and New Zealand ever approved DTC drug marketing, but the ads show up everywhere US television is broadcast, which is most of the world. In many countries, they run as filler because local advertisers do not have enough money to buy all the spots.

Here is how the system fits together: After the corporations fund and organize biased disease studies that claim a drug works, they put out press releases about how common and devastating the ailment is. The charities disease-monger, and in the US, DTC ads hawk the purported cures. Prescribing guidelines contrived by bought-off academics add fuel to the fire.

For example, GlaxoSmithKline combined press releases about social anxiety with aggressive direct-to-consumer marketing about how Paxil relieved it. They never mention that the drug creates intolerable restlessness in several percent of users and that they occasionally kill themselves. In 2004, New York attorney general Eliot Spitzer sued GlaxoSmithKline. Internal documents obtained at discovery showed that the company leaders were aware of Paxil's tendency to cause suicide. Implausibly, in 2020 the FDA still approves Paxil for social anxiety.

CHAPTER 10

DIRTY TRICKS DRIVE SALES

The promise given was a necessity of the past; the word broken is a necessity of the present.

— Niccolo Machiavelli, *The Prince* (1511)

Healthcare is not a free market. Gaming the licensing and patent system creates monopolies and can raise prices even for older drugs. Artificial shortages of vital medications increase their cost. Stalling in court with imaginative lawsuits lengthen patent monopolies. Litigation is also used to intimidate any individual or corporation that stands in a company's way. Lawyers' bills are modest expenses when a drug's revenues are in the billions.

Tampering with markets is business as usual. In 2001, several of the world's largest drug companies, led by Hoffmann-La Roche, conspired in a massive criminal price-fixing cartel to raise prices of their supplements and vitamins. A *New York Times* article reported:

The scope of the conspiracy boggles the mind. For a full decade, top executives at some of the world's largest drug companies met secretly in hotel suites and at conferences. When Federal investigators were closing in, they moved to the homes of high-level European executives... they carved up world markets and carefully orchestrated price increases, in the process defrauding some of the world's biggest food companies, including Kellogg, Coca-Cola, and Nestle... It was… the most pervasive and harmful criminal antitrust conspiracy ever uncovered.

Another strategy is to file patents to tie up competing products with lawsuits. These work even if the suits get lost, because delays based on patents prolong the period that drugs keep their profitable monopoly. Filing a patent costs $20,000, which is nothing for drug companies, and there is no limitation on the numbers filed. One company submitted 1300 for a single drug. Even generic prices can sometimes be kept high using the patent system or some other technique, as the following stories show.

EpiPen is a 30-year-old patented appliance used to inject adrenaline for the emergency treatment of an allergic reaction at home. The company that bought the device's patent increased its price over a few years from $100 to more than $600, and then to $2400 (generics are available at publication date for $300). The CEO's yearly compensation went from $2.5 to $18.9 million. This would not have been possible without insurance reimbursement. It made the news, but since few pay cash, the outcry was muted.

Insulin is arguably the most vital medication in all medical care. People with type I "insulin dependent" diabetes need it each day to stay alive. The developers sold the rights to it to a university for $1 because they did not believe patenting such a critical drug was ethical. It has been off-patent for over 75 years.

Thirty years ago, insulin manufactured from pigs or cows was less than a dollar a vial. Since then, two new generations of the drug were created in the laboratory and patented.

Manufacturers tripled the prices in the decade before 2016, from about $231 to $736 a year. Pork and beef insulin are no longer available in the US.

There are 1.25 million people in the US who have type 1 diabetes, and 96 percent of the insulin used is the expensive type, now costing about $300 for a ten cc bottle. Those without insurance spend as much as $500 a month on insulin. For some, this means struggling to buy enough to stay alive. Insulin rationing has caused fatalities. Some uninsured diabetics have bought their insulin abroad.

The manufacturers claimed that each new kind was superior. But many patients are switching back to the first generation lab-made drugs because they are just as good as the latest and far cheaper. Despite using only 15 percent of the world's insulin, we pay nearly half the total price. This is drugmaker price gouging, use of monopoly, and possible collusion.

Colchicine is a two-centuries-old medication that relieves painful gouty attacks. When a federal law was passed to encourage studying older drugs, a small company did some research that confirmed what we already knew—it helped gout. The FDA allowed them to patent it for seven years, and ordered the generic colchicine off the market. The company then jacked up the pill's price to more than $5 each, and was sold for $800 million. Thanks to litigation by generic manufacturers, colchicine is now available again in a cheaper form.

Seconal (secobarbital) was patented in 1934 and has been generic for many decades. It should cost pennies. The traditional use was for sleep, but recently it became one of the best-accepted drugs for physician-assisted suicide. In early 2015, Valeant, which purchased the medication from the prior owner, increased the price of the fatal dose to $3000.

Albendazole, the traditional pinworm treatment, is now $100 per pill or $1200 for a course of therapy. An entire family typically gets pinworms all at once from one kid, so this gets expensive. Amedra Pharmaceuticals, the sole US manufacturer, raised the price because they realized they had no competitors. The US yearly spending for this drug went from $100,000 in 2008 to $7.5 million in 2013, and there was no worm epidemic. It is still available for $1 a pill in Canada.

A very different drug was promoted similarly. The old generic antibiotic doxycycline went from 6.3 cents to $3.36 per pill between 2012 and 2014. Its manufacturer took advantage of another temporary near-monopoly situation.

Fluorouracil (5-FU): Phil is a 66-year-old friend with "actinic keratoses" on his face. Dermatologists claim these are precancerous and say that their treatment is imperative. Phil's skin doctor told him to rub the 5-FU solution on the spots for a few weeks. When he did this in the past, the generic prescription for a small bottle of this 30-year-old drug cost $80.

This time, his dermatologist gave him a special order, which the pharmacist billed to Medicare. There was no charge to the patient, so he thought all was well. A few months later, he realized Medicare and his supplemental insurance had paid $2000 for the tiny quantity of 5-FU. He speculated the drugmaker gave his dermatologist some favor or kickback to prescribe the proprietary medicine, which was identical to the old one.

Chloramphenicol was invented in 1947, and it was considered a wonder drug. It killed nearly all bacteria and was initially thought safe. By the early 1960s, it was heavily advertised for almost any minor illness and was used in a "shotgun" fashion for millions of Americans. Doctors knew they were treating mostly viral illnesses, which would not respond to antibiotics, but they knew of no dangers. There were alternatives, including doing nothing.

Within a few years, chloramphenicol was proven to cause liver and kidney damage and, in a few cases, death from aplastic anemia, which is complete blood cell suppression. Others got leukemia or other serious problems. Because it was prescribed so promiscuously, thousands likely died. Parke-Davis, the producer, marketed it even after they knew about the fatalities.

Although this was clear by the 1960s, when the FDA tried to exercise control, the company ignored them and continued to advertise aggressively. But once the drug went off patent in 1966 and became less profitable, the marketing stopped, and sales declined. No-one went to jail. The CEO responsible, Harry Loynd, commented, "If we put horse manure in a capsule, we could sell it to 95 percent of these doctors."

Ironically, since chloramphenicol was later used sparingly, resistant bacteria never developed. When patients have multi-drug resistant infections now, chloramphenicol is still an option, and it usually works.

Aricept is another wild story. This controversial Alzheimer's drug grossed $2 billion a year and was due to go off-patent in 2010. It was available in 5 and 10 mg strengths. Four months before the license expired, the company patented a 23 mg pill. Since the 5 and 10 mg pills could not be combined to make 23 mg, sales of the purportedly new formulation took off.

The FDA's scientists had internally recommended against approval of this hoax, but their chief overruled them, allowing three more years of profiteering. It was all techni-cally within the rules, but to observers, it looked like bribery.

The companies price HIV drugs outrageously, even in developing countries. Recently, some African nations had HIV rates thought by some sources to be above 30 percent. If this were true, they faced annihilation. GlaxoSmithKline (GSK) refused to allow other companies to manufacture their patented AZT (azidothymidine) anti-retroviral treatment for HIV. They claimed this would "compromise future drug discovery." They lowered their prices only after a worldwide outcry.

Daraprim: The media dubbed Martin Shkreli "the most

hated man in America" when he increased the price of this
drug from $13 to $750 per pill. This is a second-line treatment
of toxoplasmosis, a relatively common parasitic disease. It is
seldom serious, but for those with AIDS or cancer, it can be
life threatening without treatment. Daraprim is not a
frequently used drug, but because of this monopoly situation,
the manufacturer could ask any price. Ironically, Shkreli went
to jail later for securities fraud, not price gouging.

Claritin: Schering-Plough's patent for the drug was due to
expire, so they sued the new generic manufacturer that was
about to release the drug. They made the claim that the generic's FDA applications were incomplete. This had no merit,
and as expected, the lawsuit was lost. But since revenue for
Claritin was $2 billion a year, they recouped the entire $5
million in legal fees every single day the case delayed Claritin
from going off-patent. This routine practice keeps a generic
off the market with an automatic 30-month delay, and it is
business as usual.

"Pay-to-play" is a related strategy. After the patent period
expires, and another company files for a generic application,
just like the above case, the patent holder sues. They again
claim there is a technical problem with the generic's FDA
paperwork. Instead of going to court, however, they settle.
The generic company agrees to delay production if the
current patent-holder pays them. Regulators realize this pay-
to-play costs consumers billions of dollars every year and
have attempted to regulate it. The rules have become progressively more complex. The game is ongoing despite attention
from the Federal Trade Commission in the US and others in
the EU.

Drugs for rare diseases, such as certain metabolic disorders or unusual forms of cancer, are often in the news because
industry raises their prices to fantastical levels. These "specialty" medications are two percent of prescriptions *but are
now 30 percent of drugmakers' revenues*. The corporate strategy

is to publish in the *NEJM*, and the buyers will come. These diseases are so uncommon that there may not be enough patients to do proper studies to decipher whether the medications work.

To get a feel for this, look at the top-earning drugs sold in 2017. There was one cholesterol medication on the list and a new, expensive insulin. This top seller list is no longer made up of familiar antidepressants and blood-sugar-lowering drugs. These new "specialty" medications get approved because of pressure on the FDA. Among other arguments, the corporations say, "Without this drug, we will be empty-handed." An empty-handed doctor is apparently intolerable.

Tampering with anti-nausea drugs: Compazine and droperidol are $3 a dose, generic medications used to treat nausea. Here is the story of how they were removed from the marketplace to encourage sales of Zofran, an expensive alternative.

In the early 2000s, Compazine suddenly disappeared from the US, and shortages have been frequent ever since. Other countries can get all they want. Droperidol had a black-box warning slapped on it in 2001. A new study showed that the drug caused serious cardiac rhythm disturbances, *torsades-de-pointes,* and QT prolongation. When critics examined the data, they discovered that the doses used in the trial were fifty (50) times what is ordinarily used. At these doses, the drug was toxic to the heart. The world champion academic fraudster Yoshitaka Fujii had a hand in this study. He made his reputation in 2012 when he was forced to retract 183 papers because of faked research.

Zofran, costing $150 per dose, has remained available. By 2006, its sales were $1.3 billion globally (it went off patent in 2007). Thirty years of experience with droperidol was disregarded. The black-box warning from 2001 survives in 2020, and Compazine is still hard to find.

GlaxoSmithKline (GSK) promoted Zofran for pregnant

women. After a Danish study showed double the risk of fetal heart defects in babies of mothers taking it, GSK paid a $1 billion criminal settlement in 2013 for allegations of off-label marketing. The total amount they paid was $3 billion, and this included issues with other drugs. This price was affordable because Glaxo's gross revenues were $39 billion that year. Zofran's cost in the US is still $10 per intravenous dose and $23 for each pill (2017). They are 75 cents in New Zealand.

In an American-style business deal, Glaxo agreed to give a Korean company exclusive rights to market the original drug there if they would keep the generics off the market. Korea's regulator, the National Health Insurance Service (NHIS), fined GSK and the Korean drugmaker over four million dollars.

None of these medications are very active anyway, at least according to Cochrane reviews. They examined 737 studies, and the drugs only helped one in four people with their nausea. The expensive ones were no more effective than the cheap ones, and the side effects were all about the same. But some emergency physicians still believe Zofran works the best and say they cannot do without it.

————

MORE DIRTY TRICKS:

Other mysterious drug shortages have inflated prices for decades. I ran a surgical center, so I watched this. Propofol, a sedation drug, was hard to get for a while, and our wholesaler gouged us for the generics. At first, we believed the excuses. There were bacterial contamination issues in some factories, and Teva, the manufacturer, shut these down.

A Las Vegas surgicenter contaminated single-use Propofol bottles with hepatitis virus, then infected patients when they used them more than once. Baxter, the wholesaler, paid a $144 million settlement, and Teva lost a $356 million jury award to one of these people. They stopped making the drug for a few years after this.

Later, lidocaine, adrenaline, and even saltwater (saline) became harder to get, and their prices shot up. This was supposedly because of a Puerto Rico factory destroyed in a hurricane. This also affected Robinul (glycopyrrolate), a drug which keeps patients from producing too much saliva and choking during surgery. Then, in 2018, instead of buying adrenaline inexpensively in 20 cc vials, my clinic was forced to buy single one cc glass vials at ten times the price per volume. These shortages persisted on and off, but we did not hear about them happening in other countries.

Intimidation using lawsuits: Dr. Nancy Oliveri at the University of Toronto was a lead researcher in a study of a drug used to treat thalassemia major, which is a severe anemia. Apotex funded the research, and she signed confidentiality agreements. When the drug trials were underway, her team discovered a critical health issue. She wanted to inform other researchers so they could warn patients who were taking the drug. Apotex refused permission.

She consulted with lawyers and her ethics committee, who said she had a higher duty to her patients than to the company, and that the contracts were unenforceable. Apotex attempted to silence her by canceling her part of the study. They also sued her, but fortunately, the Canadian state malpractice insurance paid for her defense, even though the issue was not malpractice. She could not have afforded her attorneys otherwise. While this was happening, she performed liver biopsies on her patients and found continued damage.

Defamatory anonymous letters were sent to various staff members at her hospital. Despite her international reputation, she lost her job as chief of the abnormal hemoglobin program. DNA found on the letters proved they came from a physician working for Apotex. The University of Toronto eventually reinstated her.

Strategies used to suppress unfavorable research: Boots Pharmaceutical owned Synthroid, a patented synthetic thyroid, in the mid-1990s. They commissioned a study at the University of California San Francisco (UCSF) to prove their product's superiority to the generic drugs. The study found no difference between the generics and Synthroid. The UCSF scientists sent the paper for publication, but the journal had trouble finding experts who would review it. They all said they had a financial relationship with Boots.

Then, just before publication, the company invoked a contractual gag clause and suppressed the work for four years. UCSF fought to preserve its academic integrity but Boots threatened it with lawsuits. Eventually, Boots was bought and became Boots/Knoll. The new company published the data using ghostwriters, who claimed it proved Synthroid was superior to the generics.

When the truth came out in the *Wall Street Journal*, Boots/Knoll was forced to back down but continued to print distortions. Experts at UCSF estimated that the country wasted $350 million on expensive, patented Synthroid every year that the delays concealed the study information.

In 2016, after industry lobbying, Congress limited the DEA's power to control drug wholesalers' importation of opioids. Previously, the DEA could freeze a company's shipments if they thought it was an imminent danger to the community. This might stop massive purchases of drugs deemed dangerous. The DEA had been fighting for years to maintain this authority, but after industry lobbying, Congress passed the bill.

The chief of the DEA's Office of Diversion Control, Joe Rannazzisi, was a whistleblower. He said that the change destroyed the regulatory oversight of drug wholesalers, and as a result, Cardinal Health, McKesson, and Amerisource-

Bergen were now pumping opioids into retail pharmacies with impunity. He said that the crack epidemic was inconsequential compared to addictive prescriptions.

Gøtzsche describes the pharmaceutical industry's kickbacks, bribery, bullying, and intimidation:

> *The centrepiece of the US Organized Crime Control Act from 1970 is the Racketeer Influenced and Corrupt Organizations Act (RICO). Racketeering is the act of engaging in a certain type of offence more than once. The list of offences that constitute racketeering includes extortion, fraud, federal drug offences, bribery, embezzlement, obstruction of justice, obstruction of law enforcement, tampering with witnesses, and political corruption. Big pharma does so much of this all the time that there can be no doubt that its business model fulfils the criteria for organised crime.*

> — *Deadly Medicines and Organised Crime* (2013)

Everyone, including the regulators, profits from this activity except taxpayers and patients. The industry is happy to pay the fines, payoffs, criminal settlements, or whatever they are, as long as money continues to fall out of the sky from third-party payers. Prosecutors get publicity for the arrangements and congratulations for supposedly doing their job.

Lawyers, legislators, lobbyists, physicians, researchers, and publishers are all on the take and collect their share. The insurance companies preside over the scene like arms manufacturers. They are indifferent to who gets shot—or in this case, how much it all costs. Their take is right off the top of the entire pile of loot. The pattern has been the same for decades. The drugs almost all stay on the market, new ones come out with regularity, and profits grow every year.

We know all about these firms. Roche made its money selling heroin illegally in the US and addicted many patients

to Valium and Librium while claiming they were not addictive. They market the practically worthless Tamiflu, making
billions of dollars.

Merck concealed the cardiovascular harms of its rheuma-
tology drugs, which caused many deaths. Pfizer paid $2.3
billion for illegal marketing (which included kickbacks) of
four drugs and signed a "corporate integrity agreement" as
part of the agreement with prosecutors. It was a record settlement, but GSK beat it in 2018 when they paid $3 billion. Since
Pfizer had paid up and sworn off ill-deeds three times before,
it is unlikely they will do any better now. Peter Gøtzsche
concludes:

> **In the United States, big pharma beat all other industries in
> terms of crimes.** *They have more than three times as many serious
> or moderately serious law violations as other companies, and this
> record holds also after adjustment for company size. Big pharma
> also has a worse record than other companies for international
> bribery and corruption and for criminal negligence in the unsafe
> manufacture of drugs.*
>
> — *DEADLY MEDICINES AND ORGANISED CRIME*, 2013

These corporations are much better financed, organized,
and influential than the regulators. I wonder if they are more
powerful than governments.

CHAPTER 11

OPIOIDS AND "PAIN MANAGEMENT"

I'll tell you why I like [the cigarette business]. They cost a penny to make. Sell for a dollar. It's addictive. And there's a fantastic brand loyalty.

— WARREN BUFFETT

INTRODUCTION. By 2019, opioids were killing approximately 50,000 US citizens a year, up from 8,000 in 1999. This is more deaths than firearms (33,000), breast cancer (41,000), HIV (15,000), or motor vehicle accidents (37,000). In 2018-2019, the total fatalities exceeded our combined combat deaths in Iraq, Vietnam, and Afghanistan. Until recently, prescription rather than street opioids caused the most deaths. The per capita fatalities differ in each state, suggesting that local factors such as enforcement, economics, and education may contribute.

Street opioids and prescription opioids are chemically identical. This class includes heroin, which is illegal, plus morphine, methadone, Vicodin, fentanyl, and Demerol, which all have recognized medical uses, but are also sought illegally. OxyContin (oxycodone) is another prescription that has the street name of "Oxy." Purdue Pharma, the patent owner, told the world it was safe. They distributed it widely and made billions of dollars. They marketed it with free samples, the same method the drug cartels use, but the dealers, to their credit, never claimed their product was harmless.

Background: These opioids are effective pain relievers, traditionally used for cancer, heart attacks, severe injuries, and post-surgical pain. Opium, made from a flower, was the first of these drugs and has been used for thousands of years. Morphine was derived from opium in the early 1800s and heroin from morphine in 1874. These three plus codeine are derived from plants. They are the *opiates.* The other drugs, along with modern codeine, are manufactured in the laboratory.

Side effects include sleepiness, nausea, low blood pressure, and constipation. With continued use, patients become tolerant, which means they need higher and higher doses to get the same effect. There is a withdrawal syndrome that is not life threatening, but involves several days of terrific discomfort. The symptoms include sweating, muscle aches, nausea, vomiting, sleeplessness, restlessness, anxiety, diarrhea, and high blood pressure.

Anyone who uses opioids for prolonged periods can get this withdrawal, but addiction is different and much worse. This means users cannot stop the drugs. "Junkie" behavior is the usual result. This runs the gamut from relationship destruction up to entering a criminal lifestyle to get enough money for the next "fix." These basics have been well-known for more than a century.

Overdose deaths happen because of stopped breathing. When users combine opioids with other sedatives or alcohol, the risk is much higher. Narcan (naloxone) is an antidote that reverses opioid effects and can save an overdose victim if given before they suffocate. It lasts a shorter time than most opioids, so people receiving it must be watched for several hours to be sure they keep breathing. The drug is now over-the-counter and available at Walgreen's in 35 states and even many high schools.

Although naloxone has been available for over fifty years and is generic, the drugmakers have found a way to price gouge. They patented a nasal spray device that costs $150 for a two-pack. Another pharmaceutical company created an injection system in 2016 and jacked the price up from $690 to $4500. It was designed to be carried around by addicts for emergencies. The company rushed it through a perfunctory FDA approval process without the usual study. Dr. Katz's comment about this is: *Most of these addicts are barely functional, and this pricey medication is provided by state support. Having naloxone as a psychological margin of safety encourages addicts to abuse higher and riskier doses.*

The causes of addiction are unclear. Most people are not very vulnerable and do not search for more drugs when their pain stops. They can become tolerant, however. They then need larger and larger doses to treat pain, and they get withdrawal symptoms. These people are "dependent," but can withdraw from the drug whenever they want.

Others are susceptible to addiction and get hooked right away. Jason Smith, an addict, described his initial experience after a Demerol shot for back pain when he was 17: "That first hit. There's nothing like it in the natural world. I was in love. This feeling? I didn't want it to stop. I wanted to feel this way forever. And ever. The shame. The self-hatred. The guilt. It disappeared."

For 15 years, he was beaten up, was in and out of jail, and did "dirty, conniving, manipulative, inhumane s***" to scam people out of the money to buy his drugs. He was always looking for another Fentanyl patch to suck on. He only used prescriptions and never heroin from the street[1].

What percentage of people are vulnerable? A 2014 study in *BMJ*, "Rates and Risk Factors for Prolonged Opioid Use After Major Surgery," followed 39,000 post-surgical patients who had never used opioids. Only three percent remained on the medication for over 90 days.

A 2017 survey of 36,000 surgery patients who used these drugs for the first time revealed that five to six percent stayed on them long after their recovery. A history of smoking, depression, or abuse of alcohol or drugs increased the risk. The surgery and pain intensity had no relationship to prolonged usage. Another trial from 2006 to 2015 studied a million insured patients whose doctors gave them opioids for the first time. Usage persisted in about five to thirty percent of them. The ones taking larger quantities during their illness were more likely to have long-term addiction.

Addicts or pain patients can sometimes take over ten times the ordinary dose, which would be fatal for the uninitiated. Hydrocodone, which is Norco or Vicodin, is the same strength per milligram as morphine, so a hundred of the 10 mg tablets is 1000 mg. Some people work up to taking this much "morphine equivalent" every 24 hours. A dose of 600 mg a day is not unusual. This would stop the breathing and kill anyone not accustomed to the drug. Norco and Vicodin are a combination of the opioid and Tylenol (acetaminophen). Since physicians know that thirty of the 325 mg Tylenol tablets in one day can be fatal, this limits prescribing.

"Opioid hyperalgesia" is closely related. This describes people who have increased sensitivity to pain after chronic use. For example, my patient Sally had a hysterectomy. Her gynecologist prescribed Percocet, an opioid, to deal with her pain. He continued giving her the medication for months instead of stopping it after a week or two. She finally weaned herself off the drug without help. Later, when I performed a minor surgery for her, she suffered several months of severe pain and required opioids. If her gynecologist had not over-prescribed, she would likely have been less sensitive to this pain.

HOW THE DISASTER DEVELOPED

Before the mid-1990's, doctors prescribed opioids carefully and in limited quantities for disease-related pain. But in 1990, *Scientific American* published "The Tragedy of Needless Pain." It advocated looser prescribing: "Contrary to popular belief... morphine taken solely to control pain is not addictive. Yet patients worldwide continue to be under-treated and to suffer unnecessary agony."

After this, the indications for these drugs was broadened to include many types of acute and chronic pain. By 2001, the FDA was pressured to sanction broader prescribing, and they instituted formal guidelines to achieve this. The Joint Commission (then known as the Joint Commission on Accreditation of Healthcare Organizations or JCAHO) issued a mandate to treat pain more aggressively.

Purdue Pharma is a multi-billion dollar company privately owned by the Sackler family. It bears a heavy share of the blame for today's crisis. The company claimed their OxyContin did not create tolerance, did not make users high, and had less than a one percent addiction rate.

Purdue's marketing blew up nationwide opioid sales. They paid for 20,000 seminars to teach doctors the new treatment guidelines. Forty of these were all-expense-paid, including airfare. They made a $100,000 donation to the Federation of State Medical Boards for materials to educate doctors about the pain problem. Tracing other monies is harder, but Purdue likely gave millions to influence policy in various ways.

Pain became the "fifth vital sign." New standards of care statements soon commanded providers to ask every patient about it as they checked the heart rate, blood pressure, respiration, and temperature. If doctors did not prescribe enough opioids, their state medical boards might discipline them.

Hospitals might suffer adverse publicity from pain advocacy groups.

Purdue sent hundreds of representatives to thousands of doctors' offices, targeting primary care physicians who had no prior training in pain management. They gave away dinners, free bottles of samples, and much more. They focused on poverty areas with Medicaid patients whose medications were free through the program.

Purdue also abducted or sometimes manufactured agendas for charity groups. For example, the American Chronic Pain Association (ACPA) has industry funding that included Purdue until recently. The American Pain Foundation disbanded in 2012, probably destroyed by terrible publicity. The American Pain Society (APS) is now considering bankruptcy because their credibility has also been shredded. They received tens of thousands of dollars of industry sponsorship for their annual conference, and Pfizer paid for their grant funding.

News stories saying that 100 million Americans live with pain were everywhere. Since pharmaceutical industry sources promoted this number, it was discredited.

Purdue Pharma gave $3 million to Harvard's Mass General Hospital to rename its pain center the Purdue Pharma Pain Center. As part of the deal, the drugmaker supplied clinical education coursework for pain management standards. These details became public when hundreds of entities, including entire states, sued Purdue.

The nation was soon swimming in OxyContin. It was cheap, available everywhere, and readily used by crushing, chewing, snorting, or even injecting. Exposures at parties or through loose prescribing by doctors operating out of "pill mills" uncovered more and more vulnerable individuals. Purdue and other pharmaceutical companies exposed an entire generation of Americans to the drugs, and the susceptible ones became addicted. At first, it was cheap and available.

Purdue was the ringleader, but it was only responsible for about three percent of the oxycodone and hydrocodone sold in the US between 2006 and 2012. The big distributors, McKesson Corp., Walgreens, Cardinal Health, Amerisource-Bergen, CVS, and Walmart sold seventy-five percent. Johnson and Johnson was also heavily involved. They were ordered in 2019 to pay $571 million for their part addicting just a single state, Oklahoma. They sold opioid products to Purdue and also funded fake advocacy groups.

In 2020, plaintiffs bankrupted the US division of Mallinck-rodt, the largest single generic producer, with a $1.6 billion settlement. Its overseas affiliates are still thriving, however.

When the wave of overdoses caught national attention, prescription supplies tightened, prices went up, and people who couldn't afford "legitimate" opioids used heroin because it was cheaper. Dealers often sold this right outside "legitimate" pain clinics. Addicts did not need needles because they could smoke it.

Mexican dealers developed a sophisticated distribution and marketing system into the US, including free delivery to the customer. Joaquin Guzman (El Chapo), a billionaire drug lord now in a US prison, was the most famous of the leaders who orchestrated it. Just like Purdue, his dealers offered free samples—the first taste, as the addicts say. But they could never have been as successful as they were without the massive demand created by prescriptions. Soon, hundreds of thousands were dying. The New Hampshire chief medical examiner could not handle performing so many autopsies on young overdose patients, so he quit and entered the priesthood.

Federal prosecutors sued Purdue Pharma, who confessed to their criminal acts in 2007 and settled for $600 million. Three of their top administrators pleaded guilty to criminal charges and paid $34.5 million in fines. No-one went to jail. Purdue designed the settlement to protect itself from new lawsuits, but Kentucky, Ohio, New Hampshire, Tennessee, Oklahoma, and thousands of individual plaintiffs pressed on.

Purdue could afford the litigation for over a decade because its total OxyContin sales through 2019 were $35 billion. But by the fall of that year, the plaintiffs forced it into bankruptcy. The Sackler descendants who still privately own Purdue are also being sued, and as of the publication date, they agreed to contribute $3 billion to the settlement. Between 2008-2017, as the opioid crisis worsened, they withdrew $10.7 billion from the corporation and moved the money into Swiss and other foreign accounts. The plaintiffs are still after them.

———

TREATMENTS

Addicts are more stable and cause less trouble when they can get drugs legally. Methadone is a 24-hour opioid that has been available in Germany since 1937. In the 1960s, it began to be used as a heroin substitute to treat addiction long term. To prevent resale of the methadone, addiction clinics provide it in liquid form to be swallowed on the spot. More recently, short-term tablet prescriptions have become available. Taking this drug is preferable to a user cycling through short-acting injectable street opioids and having withdrawals every few hours. The clinics have used this cheap drug for decades.

Methadone has drawbacks, such as unsanctioned use, although addicts do not like it as much as heroin. Most users are unemployable. The addiction continues and kicking it is much worse than heroin or OxyContin. These require less than a week, but methadone takes many weeks.

Buprenorphine, an opioid that has effects lasting three days, was first used to treat addicts in the 1990s. It causes less sleepiness than methadone, so some people can work while taking it. In 2002, a pharmaceutical company combined it with naloxone, the opioid antagonist that counters opioid effects, to create Suboxone, a patented drug. This is used as an opioid substitute that addicts take chronically as a replacement drug. It was designed to be tough to abuse. If addicts dissolve it in water and inject it, the naloxone component causes an unpleasant withdrawal.

The corporations price Suboxone extravagantly. By 2013, its annual sales were $1.55 billion, more than Viagra and Adderall combined. They market it for use over a year or longer, and since it is severely addictive, this is the near-universal outcome. The longer a drug lasts, the longer the withdrawal, and buprenorphine often requires months of withdrawal. Waves of severe depression often accompany the usual opioid-induced nausea, anxiety, muscle pains, sleep disturbance, and abdominal cramps.

MORE RECENT HISTORY

Our addiction problems have become progressively worse. Over two million Americans were dependent on opioids in 2015. That year, doctors in the US gave one person in three a prescription for opioids, ninety-five million total. This was more than all the tobacco users. In 2016, 64,000 died in the US from drug overdoses, mostly from opioids. That year, the US used 80 percent of the world's opioids and took 99 percent of the total Vicodin.

Overdoses were not a daily event when I worked in emergency rooms in the 1980s. By 2014, opioid consumption caused 1.27 million emergency visits and hospitalizations in the US, 60 percent more than 2005. A CDC report said suspected opioid overdoses increased 30 percent between 2016 and 2017.

Street and prescription opioids are Siamese twins, each

fueling the other's growth. Heroin is a sideshow compared to the prescriptions. But supply grew to meet demand, as OxyContin and its relatives became more regulated and pricey. In a 2014 survey of people in opioid treatment, 94 percent said they used heroin only because prescription opioids were too expensive and hard to get. Pharmaceutical opioid sales, overdose death rates, and substance-use treatment hospitalizations increased in lockstep from 1999 to 2008. (*NEJM*, 2016).

Fentanyl, the nightmarish gift from the drug industry, is now primarily made in illegal drug labs. This short-acting synthetic opioid is 50 to 100 times stronger than morphine and 30-50 times more potent than heroin. Tiny doses may produce a high, an overdose, or even a fatality. It is sometimes mixed with or mistaken for heroin. This confusion has caused many deaths. Another hazard is that reversing an overdose requires large doses of Narcan. In 2016, black-market fentanyl surpassed prescription opioids as the most common cause of overdose death in the United States. Sources were mainly China and India, and the drugs were often transported through Mexico.

America has a homegrown supply. In July 2017, six senior executives and managers from Insys Therapeutics pleaded guilty to paying kickbacks to doctors to induce them to prescribe their fentanyl spray Subsys. As revealed by internal whistleblowers, the company gave physicians cash, dinners, and sometimes even offered corporate prostitutes. The company encouraged excessive doses and fraudulent insurance billing. One physician prescribed over $3 million worth of patches. For a single patient, Medicare paid $250,000 for eighteen prescriptions in fourteen months. She died of an overdose.

In October 2017, prosecutors arrested the 76-year-old billionaire owner and majority shareholder John Kapoor for leading this "nationwide conspiracy." They found him and four other executives guilty in 2019. The sentence was 66 months in prison and a fine of $225 million, which must have been lunch money for him. Insys was forced to admit to the kickback scheme and went into bankruptcy.

The Chinese are the primary suppliers for our street fentanyl. Because it is so concentrated, dealers mail large doses in tiny packages internationally with little chance of interception. We are to blame along with the Chinese. They are just responding to the demand we created. The West used opium as a weapon against them in the 1800s, and this is a reversal.

––––––

PAIN TREATMENTS

Most pain is self-limited if never treated with opioids. Given what we know, I have a hard time conceiving that any physician would prescribe these drugs for more than a few weeks after an auto accident or use them long-term for back pain. Even worse, why would any physician increase the dose for tolerance if the patient did not have cancer? But opioid disasters are everywhere because of the persistent idea that we must treat all pain.

My experience with post-operative cosmetic surgery patients is that they rarely need heavy drugs. When used, they help for a few days to a week at most. After that, nausea, confusion, and constipation are worse than any remaining pain. I encourage our healthy post-operative patients to take two 200 mg Motrin and two 500 mg Tylenol three to four times a day for a few days. If they insist on more, I give them ten of the 5 mg Norco, the Tylenol-opioid combination. When taking this, I instruct them to avoid regular Tylenol to avoid getting too much.

"Pain doctors" were responsible for much of this problem, and "addiction specialists" are stuck dealing with it.

Through the 1980s, physicians were careful about the type and amount of opioids prescribed. They feared addicting patients and being criticized by colleagues. The new prescribing guidelines emboldened entrepreneurs, however, and pain centers started appearing on every street corner. Lately, they have been closing down.

Behind closed doors, pain doctors and their staff agree. They say, "Most of my patients are addicts, and I hate working here." They know that part of their work has devolved into drug dealing.

The more optimistic side of this story is that addiction physicians have recently been managing the problem better. Their usual plan is to taper the opioids over months. They try to avoid Suboxone because of the terrific addiction and terrible withdrawal. Sensible laws initially allowed only 30 Suboxone patients per doctor, but this was liberalized to 100 or 275 if physicians met certain conditions.

Kaiser Permanente of Southern California is serious about pain management. They gradually reduce their pain patients' doses down to 100 mg or less of opioid equivalent a day. Their doctors are on salary and have no perverse incentive to increase procedures or office visits.

I interviewed several pain specialists. The ones in private practice need not advertise because there is an avalanche of patients in their waiting rooms. I saw grandmothers and other people who looked exactly like the people found in any internist's office. They never took street drugs—their physicians had addicted them.

Some observers, including many in our ranks, claim that lax prescribing standards caused the debacle. But legislatures have recently constructed tighter controls. Since the new prescribing standards, it is harder for physicians to create an addict. In California, for example, a rule now says that we must use a databank to check nearly any medication we prescribe, including those for blood pressure and cholesterol.

This is expensive, excessive, and egregious, but it is a well-meaning attempt to introduce oversight. Our exam rooms are still full of addicts created over the past two decades. It is a painful problem for everyone.

———

PERSPECTIVE BY ABRAHAM KATZ, MD: *Dr. Yoho is in his mid-60s, and I am in my late 30s. I went to school during the era when "the tragedy of needless pain" became a concern. Based on my training, study, and experience, I believe that patients other than those with cancer and acute surgical problems may benefit from chronic opioid use. Our prescribing, however, has gone too far and is now part of the problem.*

The pendulum may have swung in the wrong direction. For example, my father had terminal cancer. During his recovery after a painful surgery, the doctors gave him 1 mg of morphine IV every 6 hours. This is an ineffective dose, and we requested that the doctors also give him Tylenol, which controlled his pain better than the tiny dose of morphine.

Opioids are the most potent medications we have for treating pain, and there are situations where they are appropriate. We must always consider alternatives first, but we should use opioids when they are necessary.

The last word by the author: Our policy of slaughtering our populace by bathing them in opioids dwarfs any complaints by legitimate pain patients. We must limit these drugs to cancer, heart attacks, severe injuries, and post-surgical pain. There are a few exceptions to this traditional approach—but they do not come to mind for me.

CHAPTER 12

EVERYONE TAKES AMPHETAMINES

We used to have a name for sufferers of ADHD. We called them boys.

— Anonymous

Background: For opioids, the deaths, addiction, and social destruction are the drug industry's fault—there is no controversy. There is now an anemic effort to fine and sometimes imprison a handful of people who were partly responsible for the death of more people than most wars.

There is no consensus, however, for the closely related situation of amphetamines and similar stimulants, possibly because there are only 10,000 US deaths a year. Doctors who are in the pockets of manufacturers still proclaim with straight faces that amphetamine-class prescriptions are worlds apart from the same drugs used for abuse. They say that we are under-medicating despite close to universal usage.

Physicians promote prescription stimulants for attention deficit hyperactivity disorder (ADHD) and other syndromes. Classroom misbehavior gets kids a quick prescription these days. Fidgeting, squirming, interrupting, forgetting, and being disorganized are the symptoms. For adults, the criteria are inattention, hyperactivity, impulsivity, and other similar issues. This has made ten percent of our children and many adults "legitimate" drug candidates.

American psychiatrists now treat ADHD with at least fifty prescription medications (listed on drugs.com). These include antidepressants, stimulants, and even anti-virals. Most are FDA Schedule II, the category that contains cocaine, Demerol, and other drugs considered the most hazardous. (Schedule I drugs have no accepted medical use.) Antidepressants and milder Schedule IV stimulants such as Provigil are also used.

The four chemically similar drugs on the table below are used to treat most of the ADHD cases. They all have similar effects and toxicities, all are Schedule II, and they are all produced by drugmakers. Psychiatrists split hairs about their differences, and patients have somewhat individual reactions, but these medications are far more alike than different.

Methamphetamine is first on the list below. It is the same chemical as the street drug "meth." It is manufactured both legally and illegally in the US. Most meth comes from Mexico. Recreational use entails uncontrolled doses that are often many times stronger than the prescriptions.

"AMPHETAMINE RELATIVES"		
Common/Trade Name:	Chemical:	Status:
1) 'Meth,' Desoxyn	methamphetamine (Mix of levo- and dextro-)	SCHED II PHARMACEUTICAL: legal in the US for ADHD and obesity Quick onset, most addictive. SCHED II ILLEGAL: "meth" is made on the street
2) Adderall	amphetamine and D-amphetamine mix	SCHED II PHARMACEUTICAL: probably stronger than the next two Obetrol brand is used for weight loss. Taken off the market, 1981. Addiction concerns. Marketed again without D-amphetamine For children.
3) Ritalin	Methylphenidate	SCHED II PHARMACEUTICAL: not an amphetamine, but similar. Like Adderall, but weaker.
4) Vyvanse/Concerta	Lisdexamfetamine dimesylate amphetamine	SCHED II PHARMACEUTICAL prodrug, much like Adderall, but weaker. Long-lasting.

THE 2020 NATIONAL SURVEY ON DRUG USE AND HEALTH estimated that in 2017, there were 1.2 million meth abusers in the US. In 2010, there were 1854 fatalities, but by 2017, the deaths had climbed to over 10,000.

———

HISTORY AND USE

The first amphetamine was discovered in Berlin in 1887, and they became widely used in the 1960s. The FDA approved them initially to treat obesity, and they saturated our society. The studios famously gave Judy Garland amphetamines and barbiturates when she was a child actor in *The Wizard of Oz*. Their goal was both to keep her slender and also to keep her going during their brutal filming schedule. She struggled with addiction her whole life and finally died of an overdose at 47.

In 1987, an American Psychiatric Association committee

voted the ADHD diagnosis into existence. This updated "minimal brain dysfunction," another vague label. This "hyperactivity" of children is the drugs' current primary indication. Through a political process involving consensus statements of experts, more diagnoses were soon concocted, and the prescriptions multiplied. Psychiatrists now regard the syndrome as a neurologic disease—but there is no physiological evidence for this, only opinion.

To promote legitimacy, psychiatry has voted names for these syndromes in and out of fashion. They give the terms gravitas by publication in the *DSM*, their diagnostic manual. However, many physicians and others have repeatedly questioned the credibility of the entire process. For example, in 1979, the FDA forbade the use of the minimal brain dysfunction name, which had created a fiction of an organic cause or a structural brain abnormality. But the psychiatrists soon replaced it.

The descriptions of hyperactive kids have mutated over the decades:

- ✪ Minimal brain damage (from the early 1960s)
- ✪ learning/behavioral disabilities
- ✪ Hyperactivity
- ✪ Hyperkinetic Reaction of Childhood (1968)
- ✪ Attention-Deficit Disorder (ADD), some with hyperactivity (1980)
- ✪ Attention-Deficit Hyperactivity Disorder (ADHD, since 1987)

Over a hundred symptoms are supposedly associated with this syndrome, including:

- ✪ Dyslexia
- ✪ Dysgraphia
- ✪ Dyscalculia
- ✪ Visual perception problems
- ✪ Dysarthria
- ✪ Hyperactivity

✪ Reduced attention span

✪ Temper tantrums

✪ Aggression

✪ Clumsiness

✪ "Vague spells."

By definition, the intellect is unaffected. The psychiatrists claim ten to twenty percent of the population has this problem.

Medication effects. These drugs slow down hyperactive kids and help some of them concentrate better. But if children take larger doses, they get high and hopped-up.

After the childhood market became saturated, drug marketers went after adults, and several of these medications were soon FDA approved for them as well. With low doses, many adults slow down, but they become more active with higher doses. These stimulants all increase heart rate, blood pressure, and temperature. Reduced appetite, weight loss, and temporary high alertness are common effects. Workers may use the amphetamine relatives to work double or triple shifts. They get them by prescription, from the street, or sometimes from their own kids.

The industry marketed a five-minute ADHD question- naire to make the diagnosis. Schoolteachers who have kids with hard-to-manage behavior often start the process. In many places, they refer the kid to a primary care doctor. Some of these physicians have been called "prescription automats" because they briefly examine the patient, then pass the drugs out like jelly beans.

If the parents refuse to let their son—boys get drugged much more often than girls—take medicine, teachers and others may pressure them. There are reports of referrals to child protective services for "non-compliant" parents. There may be threats and even occasional court orders involved, and some children have been taken away. Websites encourage parents to take legal action against their spouse or former spouse if they disagree about the need for medications. Lawyers regard this subject as legally fascinating, and it has become a topic of law reviews.

Those who doubt the benefit of the drugs have criticized this process bitterly. The youngest kids in each grade often display behavior that is not as well-controlled as their peers, and they may get diagnosed. The critics say the drugs suppress healthy childhood behaviors, particularly for boys, for the convenience and comfort of teachers, with little regard for long-term safety or efficacy.

The corporations disease-mongered the ADHD diagnosis into near-ubiquitous use, starting with the invention of the name Adderall, which sounds like "ADD for all."

———

STIMULANT HARMS

There are hundreds of reports of cardiac problems, including fatalities. Since (illegal) meth is used in higher doses, the short-term problems are more obvious. These amphetamine relatives produce depression, sleeplessness, anxiety, and sometimes delusions or even hallucinations. When this happens, doctors push other diagnoses on the kids. These include depression, bipolar, anxiety, and obsessive-compulsive disorder.

The drugs are rarely discontinued. Instead, new symptoms—or rather side effects—get treated with a variety of other medications. The worst part is that the kids become convinced that there is something permanently wrong with them, and they turn into lifetime customers of the drugmakers.

Expert opinions:

✪ Bruce Perry, leading neuroscientist and a senior fellow of the Child Trauma Academy in Houston, Texas, says that childhood hyperactivity is not a real disease. He states that there are no long-term benefits of the drugs and that no study has ever shown benefits for ADHD. He cites the animal studies that reveal brain damage.

✪ Fred Baughman describes studies showing brain atrophy (shrinkage) *The ADHD Fraud*, 2006.

✪ Richard Saul, MD, who wrote *ADHD Does Not Exist* (2014), says the drugmakers invented and promoted the whole syndrome with the collusion of psychiatrists, all for profit, ignoring the harm done to vulnerable young people. In 1987, there were 500,000 US children on the stimulants. Since then, the numbers have exploded, and now nearly five million kids are taking the drugs.

✪ Edward Hallowell wrote books and made his living promoting these drugs. He said, however, "I hate to think I have had a hand in creating that problem," and he apologized for saying they were safer than aspirin. He said that we now make ADHD diagnoses in a slipshod fashion, and he believes prescribing the drugs as "mental steroids" is wrong.

✪ Keith Connors is a psychologist and professor emeritus at Duke University who is said to have invented the stimulant treatment of children. He resurfaced in recent years, calling the use of the medications "a national disaster of dangerous proportions... The numbers make it look like an epidemic. Well, it's not. It's preposterous... a concoction [used] to justify the giving out of medication at unprecedented and unjustifiable levels." Connors woke up to the problems when he read a massive study that showed only a few percent of the children who got prescriptions had ADHD. He says he deeply regrets the way we now use the drugs.

✪ Roger Griggs was the executive for Shire Pharmaceuticals, the company that introduced Adderall in 1994. He said recently that his opinions have changed, and he believes these drugs should not be marketed because of the dangers. He says they are "nuclear bombs," to be used only under extreme circumstances, and with careful monitoring.

✪ Peter Breggin, MD, is a psychiatrist who has dedicated his career to warning about the harms of these medications. He writes:

> *Once you've given the child a stimulant medication, the child is very likely to … get euphoric, get depressed, get irritable, get angry, get upset, and that can lead to a misdiagnosis of bipolar disorder… forty years later, children started in the seventies on small doses of stimulant drugs for ADHD can end up as career mental patients… with a higher mortality rate, a higher suicide rate, a higher rate of incarceration, a higher rate of mental hospitalization, lower economic and educational success… They have increased obesity and they have atrophy of the brain.*
>
> — PSYCHIATRIC DRUG WITHDRAWAL *(2012)*

Some stimulant studies: Vibhore Prasad and others did a meta-analysis of 43 studies with 2,110 patients (2012), and concluded the stimulants made ADHD patients better. Richard Saul refuted this:

> *The review's results… were only reported as percentages on an undefined scale without standard deviations. Furthermore, the quality of the trials was poor. Two-thirds [of the trials] couldn't be included in the meta-analysis, and most had problems with missing data and didn't report an adequate randomisation method. There was a huge scope for reporting bias, and there must have been unblinding bias, as the drugs have conspicuous side effects.*
>
> — *ADHD* DOES NOT EXIST: THE TRUTH ABOUT ATTENTION DEFICIT AND HYPERACTIVITY DISORDER *(2014)*

Another example: Gonon and his team (2012) reviewed 47 research papers about ADHD published during the 1990s.

They said, "Of the top ten papers, seven claimed to verify novel hypotheses. Of these, the conclusions of six were either completely refuted or substantially weakened by subsequent investigations. The seventh has been neither confirmed nor denied."

A long-term study of over 500 children revealed stunted growth without behavior improvement. A 2018 study of nearly 600 seven to nine-year-old boys also showed ADHD medications stunted their growth—by an average of two inches.

———

THE EVOLUTION OF THE PROBLEM

ADHD diagnoses have exploded—here are the numbers. According to the American Psychiatric Association, about 8.4 percent of American children and 2.5 percent of adults now have ADHD. The CDC's (2017) number is 11 percent of the 4 to 17-year-olds. In Louisiana, the state with supposedly the highest ADHD rate, up to 50 percent of the boys in some elementary schools are diagnosed, and 93 percent of them are treated with medications.

Between 2008 and 2012, the number of Americans who took these medications rose 36%, to over 4.8 million people. Another source confirmed: prescription stimulant usage in the US doubled from 2006 to 2016. The media is constantly and breathlessly reporting figures about this "disease." Everyone seems to believe that the kids, not the doctors, have the problem.

The US uses 70 percent of the stimulants consumed world-wide (and 75 percent of all prescription drugs). ADHD is now the second most frequent long-term diagnosis for children after asthma.

These drugs now commonly are used off label for toddlers. According to the CDC, the two to five-year-olds who have ADHD have increased more than half from 2007 to 2012. By 2016, there were purportedly 388,000.

These companies have paid immense criminal settlements. Teva Pharmaceuticals, for example, had a $1.2 billion FTC settlement for "pay-to-delay" agreements to keep Adderall on patent. It is a complex and unappetizing story.

Janssen Pharmaceuticals is the maker of Concerta (another brand name for Ritalin) and a subsidiary of Johnson & Johnson. They paid $2.2 billion to settle criminal and civil charges in 2013 for the alleged promotion of several drugs for uses unapproved by the FDA, and payment of kickbacks to physicians and a long-term care pharmacy provider.

Civil litigants have also filed many personal injury and class-action lawsuits against the stimulant manufacturers, alleging childhood violence and suicidality.

I interviewed students at several Ivy League universities. They frequently use Provigil, a milder schedule IV stimulant, or sometimes one of the four schedule II drugs in the table above to study, take exams, and write papers. Many, if not most, students in these top schools use the drugs—they claim they must take them to compete. The rumors say that a third of students in Ivy League schools have a "legitimate" diagnosis. They sell their medications to their peers. A Michigan college study found that nine percent of those surveyed had current prescriptions for Adderall, and 24 percent had gotten some and used it.

The kids are familiar with these drugs, and they have preferences. For example, some like the extended-release versions best. A story I heard was, "When I take Provigil, I get constipated and pick at my skin. Adderall is much better." Another student said: "I don't socialize as much when I take Ritalin."

Drug consumption starts in prep school. Faking symptoms and getting a prescription is easy. Both the amphetamine-type medications and the opioids are readily available for sale from retirees on fixed incomes. Provigil can be purchased online without a prescription from foreign pharmacies. Parents take their kids' medications, and the kids borrow their friends.' The street price at East Coast colleges is $2 to $5 a pill for Adderall at the time of publication.

In 1991, after a lobbying effort by manufacturers, ADHD became a disability under the federal Individuals with Disabilities Education Act. Kids get extra time on tests, including the SAT. Entire families can get disability benefits sometimes.

The result is that children take less responsibility for their behavior. They may have fewer chances to learn how to control themselves, and they may have less pressure to improve because of their purported condition.

The future. Marketing researchers have seen how lucrative this industry is. One 2015 source predicted that by 2020, ADHD medications would have worldwide gross sales of $17.5 billion. *Bloomberg* reported in 2019 that the total would be $24.9 billion by 2024. The exact figures in 2020 as I publish this are unclear, but they are gloomy.

In 2014, industry developed another deliriously inclusive diagnosis: "sluggish cognitive tempo." Lilly's video describes this and recommends more drugs. Amphetamines and their relatives are now being pushed aggressively for that vast, new category: adults.

———

STREET USE

Here are the "recreational" drugs: Marijuana is the most commonly used, then the opioids, lumping together the street and prescriptions. The amphetamines are third, again counting both meth and the prescribed stimulants. In 2016, six and a half percent of all US citizens had used meth by the time they were 26 years old.

To repeat, the meth made on the streets is identical to

methamphetamine, the first of the four prescription drugs in the table above. With the higher doses typical of abuse, people get euphoric and sped-up for 8 to 24 hours. Users smoke, snort, inject, or take meth orally. Cocaine has similar effects, but it is used less because it is expensive. It only lasts about thirty minutes, so it is less harmful.

In the long run, these drugs damage body systems, including the mouth, heart, kidneys, liver, and brain. The list of chemicals used to make meth may include drain cleaner, battery acid, paint thinner, and anhydrous ammonia, which is a gas used in fertilizer and refrigerant.

Withdrawal after lengthy periods of consuming high doses produces fatigue, seizures, depression, anxiety, and insomnia. "Tweaking" is the jittery state which occurs after the drug is taken for many hours or days. Symptoms include euphoria, disturbed speech, agitation, anxiety, and sometimes paranoia with aggressiveness. Strokes occur occasionally with heavy usage. The blood pressure rises, and there is brain bleeding. Finger movements and repeated rubbing of the mouth or face are frequent and occasionally persist long term.

Emergency physicians treat people on multi-day highs who are sometimes violent and hallucinating. Psychosis, or loss of contact with reality, has been reported in 10 percent of chronic street meth users in the US and 50 percent in Japan. Symptoms like these usually go away after 5 to 7 days, but some are persistent. One study reported psychosis in 6 of 98 children who were given amphetamines for less than two years.

A common pattern is to use meth, have a psychotic episode, and then get stuck on antipsychotics for years. This happened to a friend of mine. His doctors told him he had schizophrenia and refused to help him taper off the medications. He did it himself and had a harrowing withdrawal.

Law enforcement recognizes users, manufacturers, and dealers as violent, paranoid, aggressive, delusional, and often armed. These "meth-heads" are the most unreliable and dishonest of the street drug people. They have been called coyotes because they are often homeless and prowl around looking for drugs, trying to survive. Their teeth rot, they age rapidly, and they die early.

Pseudoephedrine (Sudafed) is an over-the-counter nasal decongestant that is a critical ingredient used to make street meth. Sixteen branded US products contain it. Their yearly sales are over $600 million (2011). We import all these ingredients, and between 2005 and 2010, the volume increased by 140 percent, from 382,000 kilograms to 650,000 kilograms a year.

Congress passed a federal law in 2006 that finally required buyers to show their identification. It also created daily and monthly limits on the amount of the drug one person could buy. The manufacturers aggressively opposed these rules. Since these were already state law in most places, it did not help much, anyway. In 2007, federal law limited the importation of bulk pseudoephedrine, and we placed it behind-the-counter. This did not seem to have had much effect. There was no national movement to make it a prescription.

A third of hospitalized burn patients in some counties, such as Franklin, Missouri, are there because of meth laboratory fires. Terrifically flammable and corrosive ingredients are mixed in containers as small as a coke bottle using a method known as "shake and bake." These amateur chemists often learn their trade on a YouTube video, and may end up spending six months in a burn ward. This can cost taxpayers as much as $6000 per day.

Oregon and Mississippi passed laws that required prescriptions for pseudoephedrine compounds. There was a dramatic reduction in their meth arrests, meth treatment admissions, and even burn unit occupancy. Meth laboratory incidents nearly vanished over the short term. This was a win, but the drug manufacturers lobbied to keep other states from going down the same road.

Groups such as the National Association of State Controled (*sic*) Substance Authorities advanced the counter-narratives. They said these trends were short-term. Drug-makers and distributors heavily sponsor this group and others. This organization has a substantial website, but they misspelled their own name in the footer of their document. I speculate that they hired some semi-illiterate copywriters to promote their point of view.

The pseudoephedrine manufacturers say that importation from Mexico is now the primary problem, and that restriction of decongestant sales has little impact on meth manufacture. They are right, but I do not think it makes them less culpable for their careless sales of pseudoephedrine. Mexico has become our biggest methamphetamine supplier, and the 2017 purity is high. In return, we exported violence. Since 2006, over 200,000 drug-related killings occurred in Mexico.

THE SITUATION TODAY

Stimulants are not well accepted in other countries. France has only one amphetamine relative available, Ritalin. Only 0.46 percent of their kids take it.

Japan has substantial experience with these drugs that dates to when their chemists first synthesized meth-amphetamine in 1893. Their military used them widely in World War II. They banned or tightly controlled the medications since 1951, and the country has a "zero tolerance" policy today. The Japanese believe they are devastatingly addictive.

Although Western experts claim that ADHD is ubiquitous, the Japanese believe that it is rare or even speculative. Adderall, the amphetamine compound, is smothered with regulations, and they use Concerta, the weaker, longer-acting drug, instead. Taking these medications into the country without special permission, even for personal use, lands you in prison. Japan also bans the importation and sale of any pseudoephedrine product of over ten percent active ingredient because of their potential to be used in manufacturing.

This ADHD/stimulant frenzy follows the pattern of other patented drugs. Overwhelming marketing promotes biased industry studies that purport to show benefits. The profits with insurance reimbursement are mind-boggling.

Rabid supporters are everywhere. The journals, the drug-makers, the psychiatrists, and the academics all make money on the action. The psychiatrists' near-universal opinion is that this diagnosis is a disability that impedes success. They claim that the drugs allow drive and intelligence to emerge. In their circles, it is heresy to suggest illegitimacy.

The harms are clear, however. There are reports of brain and cardiac damage and deaths with both street and prescription stimulants. Longer-term studies show no benefit. We are encouraging both disability labeling and the use of other toxic psychiatric drugs to treat side effects.

There is no easy fix. These drugs are disastrously overprescribed, street use is a calamity, and we have no proper plan to deal with any of it.

Perspective by Dr. Katz: *As a recently trained physician, I believe this chapter has flaws. First, I do not think we should equate prescription medical use with abuse. The doses are far higher for street use. And although our medical usage is widespread, based on both my personal experience and study, I believe the positive effects of prescribed amphetamine-like drugs outweigh the harm, but we need more studies.*

Breggin confuses correlation with causation. The reason the kids received these medications makes them more likely to have problems later.

Sudafed is useful for treating allergies and sinus congestion.

I also believe that ADHD of adults is a real diagnosis, it is treat-

able with these drugs, and it is possibly under-diagnosed. Dr. Yoho's case against amphetamines appears circumstantial. He seems to believe that because so many people are taking these drugs that it is wrong.

Author's comment: My opinions are not popular with physician reviewers, who are trained to intervene. Here, this means prescribing something, anything. The studies have shown minimal or no long-term efficacy and significant long-term, permanent toxicity. This should preclude their use. The obvious damages seen with the high doses taken by street junkies are a minor problem compared to the ubiquitous usage of lower doses by nearly everyone else.

CHAPTER 13

GENERICS: GOOD, BAD, OR FAKE?

The history of the twentieth century was dominated by the struggle against totalitarian systems of state power. The twenty-first will no doubt be marked by a struggle to curtail excessive corporate power.

— ERIC SCHLOSSER *IN FAST FOOD NATION*

WE HAVE ALLOWED our patent drugmakers to gouge us so thoroughly that we can no longer afford their products. The result is that ninety percent of America's medications are now generics. Until recently, I believed that these were practically equivalent to the brand names, but it stunned me to learn I was wrong.

Generics are not exact copies of trade-name drugs. The manufacturers do not have the original recipe, and production outside the brand factories tends to be less careful. Overseas, there might be hygiene problems or extra ingredients added. These can change the way a drug works or even be harmful.

We permit new companies to manufacture drugs after the patent expires. Other companies make generics in foreign countries where patent laws are ignored. The drug's chemical name is used to market generics rather than the original trade name, and sometimes the generic drugmaker makes up their own trade name.

Lipitor generics illustrate how it works. Richard Mason (Harvard), collected thirty-six samples of this statin drug from fifteen countries and two dozen manufacturers between 2011 to 2013. Analysis proved that thirty-three had impurities that thoroughly compromised them. This is beyond atrocious, but the backstory is worse.

When the patented version of Lipitor was originally studied during its approval process, only two small groups lived longer: those who had a previous heart attack and (possibly) those with hereditary high cholesterol. This alleged success was used to support marketing to nearly anyone with slightly high cholesterol. There are now 35 million US citizens taking Lipitor. It is not just the bestselling statin, but in 2011, it was the bestselling medication of all time.

Lipitor was an ideal drug for fraudulent generic copies because the genuine item was nearly worthless. Neither the doctors, the public, the study authors, nor the writers of the two otherwise excellent resource books I used for this chapter ever understood the irony.

Although the brand-name drugmakers are guilty of many sins, they are rarely accused of poor manufacturing standards. They get so much money from the monopoly and third-party reimbursement that they can afford to make drugs accurately. Their only recent production issues have been Gilead's hepatitis C drug and a few cancer, migraine, and HIV medications.

The generics are another story. Because of our soaring drug prices, eighty percent of all US medications now originate in India or China, counting both ingredients and finished products. A 1970 Indian law allowed copying patented drugs. The only requirement was that the manufacturer had to alter some step in their process. Soon, they were producing forty percent of our generics. Some are close replicas, but others are weak, and some have extra ingredients that produce harmful effects. When doctors use weak (substandard) or ineffective (counterfeit) drugs for sick people, suffering and occasional death result. With antibiotics, weak ones breed resistant bacteria, the "superbugs."

Proper drug manufacture requires painstakingly clean and sometimes sterile chemistry. Testing and documentation at every step is the traditional way to assure quality, and this is expensive. If the makers cut corners, the savings are at least 25 percent. The horror stories about careless overseas manufacture include tablets containing bugs, glass, and hair. Inspectors have discovered facilities with bird infestations and a sterile factory in the middle of a pig farm. There are thousands of drug-making shops, and monitoring them all is impossible.

Katherine Eban in *Bottle of Lies* (2019) depicts the FDA as sluggish, grossly under-funded, understaffed, uncaring, incompetent, and sometimes corrupt. Worst of all, they are under severe political pressure to speed cheap foreign generics through the approval process. Despite this, and although we regard the Japanese and European agencies highly, the FDA is still the world leader in quality-assurance.

Their goal is to do an investigation every two years on every US and overseas manufacturing operation that makes products sold in the US. This happens domestically, but abroad they are lucky to perform one check per facility every ten years. Surprise inspections are routine in the US, but in foreign countries, the FDA allows scheduling, so managers have a few weeks to clean things up before investigators arrive. In the past, plant records were on paper, but now, computer systems pose additional difficulties for auditors.

With a visit of only five to seven days, even the most sophisticated, motivated, and aggressive inspector has trouble sorting out what is happening at a manufacturing plant. Since they are paid US government wage scales, they are rarely enthusiastic about foreign travel. Other obstacles include language and cultural barriers, bribery, threats, and even being housed in bugged hotel rooms that allow the local managers to listen to their conversations.

The FDA has comprehensive rules about drug making, and most inspectors try to enforce them. Peter Baker, a top investigator who was working in India, resorted to looking in the facilities' garbage for discarded complaint files and testing documents. He chased employees through buildings after observing them hiding records. He got into computer systems and found faked data. He caught entire rooms of people falsifying information.

The rise and fall of Ranbaxy, an Indian corporation, is Eban's major story. She quotes Dinesh Thakur, one of their employees:

> *[Ranbaxy] substituted lower-purity ingredients for higher ones ... altered test parameters so that formulations with higher impurities could be approved. They faked dissolution studies... [and] crushed up brand-name drugs... so that they could be tested in lieu of the company's own drugs. They superimposed brand-name test results onto their own ... [and] fraudulently mixed and matched data streams... [and] invented data. Document forgery was pervasive... employees backdated documents and then artificially aged them in a steamy room overnight in an attempt to fool regulators... It was common knowledge [throughout the corporation].*

He warned his superiors that their only option was a systemic overhaul. They ignored him. He quit, and he contacted the FDA in August 2005. Whistleblowers in India sometimes get murdered. Thakur's spiritual and ethical compass drove him to risk his life and career for the patients taking his company's drugs.

The FDA was clueless about Ranbaxy, but when Thakur

handed them nearly every detail, they opened a file. By 2008, three years after Thakur's first contact, they had done little. The agency only woke up when the Maryland US Attorney filed a court motion about Ranbaxy. This reported there was a "pattern of systemic fraudulent conduct by the company" and that the "violations continue to result in the introduction of adulterated and misbranded products into interstate commerce with the intent to defraud or mislead." Two weeks later, the FDA received a heads-up email that there would be a congressional investigation into why the agency had not banned Ranbaxy's products from the US. After this second warning, the FDA administrators began writing memos justifying themselves. They banned drugs coming into the US from two Ranbaxy plants but did not recall medications that were already in the US.

After Thakur left the company, his fortunes and finances declined. He initially did not understand that he could ever get paid for standing up to Ranbaxy, but years later, US class-action lawyers took the case. After arduous litigation, Thakur received $48 million. He then worked for two years on a lawsuit against the Indian federal government, claiming their broken drug regulation structure was unconstitutional there. His lawyers billed him $250,000, but the court dismissed the case after a brief hearing. His motivation was never about the money.

Ranbaxy might be an extreme case, but Eban shows that clumsy FDA oversight of foreign operations causes harmful drugs, injured patients, and corporate corruption.

More stories from Eban: GVK Biosciences was a contract research organization used by Indian firms to document their medication quality. An employee whistleblower alleged they performed routine data manipulation, and after investigation, the European Medicines Agency suspended European distribution of seven hundred drugs they had tested.

A 2014 inspection by four international regulatory agencies, including the FDA, proved that GVK committed fraud. For example, they found exact duplicate EKGs on multiple patient records. In 2016, the corporation quietly withdrew from the testing business. There were no consequences for their leaders, but the whistleblower was imprisoned in India.

Ranbaxy's standards were different for different markets. Where there was oversight, such as Europe, they sold somewhat higher quality drugs but still cheated in ways that were hard to detect. For example, they often faked expiration dates and tested one set of samples while selling others. But for Brazil, Thailand, Vietnam, Peru, Kenya, Uganda, Egypt, and other African nations, they completely fabricated the testing and manufacturing data and used lower quality ingredients.

In parts of Africa, doctors often keep supplies of patented drugs they know work. They use these for cases where the generics are not working. Because some generics are less active than the genuine thing, another strategy is to double and redouble the doses when necessary. Having an active drug is essential for gravely ill people, such as those with meningitis.

With India and China, the world's two major discount drugmakers, you get what you pay for. Each has its own unique issues.

————

INDIA HAS cheap labor and an English-speaking workforce, both significant advantages. Ramesh Venkataraman recently described the disadvantages in the *Indian Express*:

> *Ask any international businessman or investor about India, and the word "difficult" is bound to pop up.... India, despite its many obvious attractions, is seen as a tough place to do business in. Red tape and the inconsistent and arbitrary manner in which our governments have administered taxes and investment rules and*

regulations is, of course, an important reason for this sentiment.
But what polite and politically correct international investors will
not say openly is that Indians are seen as highly unethical.

The 2016 "Global Business Ethics Survey" ranked India in
the bottom three of thirteen major countries, along with
Russia and Brazil. This measures illegal activity, abuse of
ethical principles, and violations of organizational values
observed by employees. Ernst and Young's "Asia-Pacific 2017
Fraud survey" reported that 78 percent of respondents from
India said that bribery and corrupt practices are frequent.

Transparency International found 69 percent of people
surveyed said they had to pay a bribe, the highest rate in
Asia. Another article in the *HinduBusinessLine.com* explains:
"Businesses [in India] short-change customers and other businesses. Finally, a breakdown of trust boomerangs on them."
They give examples that range from tourism to financial
services to housing. Doctors take inducements as well.

These problems are petty thievery compared with ours,
however. American healthcare is systemically corrupt on a
mammoth scale, but no-one ever acknowledges it. Eban did
not understand the irony of being critical of India. Their graft
is amateurish.

India's poverty and 25 percent illiteracy rate must
contribute to their business style. On the interface between
two contrasting cultures, trust becomes tenuous and costs go
higher, sometimes in concealed ways such as poor quality.
With these obstacles, the only way to get top quality work is
the use of overbearing supervision, which is difficult from
thousands of miles away.

**The authors of *China Rx* (2019) explain the difference
between the two countries:** "India is different from China
because it is not an existential threat to the United States. It
does not have a centralized plan, designed and executed at
the highest level of government, to drive out global competi-

tors, dominate the world market, instill fear of retribution, or use its leverage to extract economic and political concessions from countries dependent on it."

The Chinese work ethic is almost religious. In theory, their culture is well-suited to the exacting manufacturing standards required for drugs. In theory, they need little supervision after a task is delegated.

Just as in India, however, many people in China are out to make a fast buck. A heparin formulation that Chinese firms sold to the US contained a synthetic ingredient, oversulfated chondroitin sulfate. The FDA speculated that the drugmaker added this substance to increase the amount of product to sell. Reactions to it were sometimes life-threatening. By 2008, there were 81 US fatalities. One man lost both his wife and son to the drug within a month.

US scientists discovered NDMA, a carcinogen once used in rocket fuel, in Chinese-made Diovan (valsartan), a blood pressure medication. In an unusually frank admission, the manufacturing company explained that this was also used to increase yields. European regulators recalled dozens of products.

Melamine is a plastic introduced into the domestic Chinese milk supplies to make them seem to contain more protein. Several hundred thousand babies fell ill, and more than ten died. Twenty-five foreign countries banned Chinese milk. The Chinese executed two leaders of the milk producers in 2009, and others involved in the scandal received lengthy prison sentences.

The first head of China's FDA-type agency took bribes to approve untested medicine. Ten deaths occurred, and China executed him in 2007. There must be more to the story, but we have no idea since it is China.

In 2015, Peter Baker, who spoke only rudimentary Mandarin, was the only FDA investigator stationed in China. He was responsible for over 400 facilities, and his experiences were similar to those he had in India. He saw ruined or vanishing audit trails, and the Chinese routinely denied him access to records and even entire facilities. They sometimes transported him to plants that were counterfeit Potemkin-village setups.

Solutions: As a stopgap, some US institutions are operating like a mini-FDA. For example, Cleveland Clinic detected reduced efficacy of certain generics after the cardiology patients who took them got sick or even died. Lab testing proved certain ones were inactive, so the doctors substituted brand-name drugs, and many patients improved. Since then, the Clinic developed a program to test generics. Other groups have followed suit.

The FDA is ineffectual. Since corporate fees pay 46 percent of their 2019 budget (the low estimate), closing dangerous manufacturing operations affects the FDA's ability to make its own payroll. And when drugs never get approved, the agency loses revenue. And although the FDA has no directive for speedy drug and device approval, Congress applies pressure to make novel things available sooner and relieve perceived shortages. The corporations leverage these perverse incentives and make the FDA's enforcement process anemic.

The following would fix our system. We know what is ineffective—attempted oversight of thousands of manufacturing facilities around the globe by this US agency. Our well-meaning traditional quality control method involves checking documents and examining processes rather than testing products.

Because drug analysis is now cheap, I propose we spend the FDA budget testing drug samples at their point of entry into our system. They have already started limited testing programs, but the budget is only a few million dollars. Since three of the US wholesalers account for 90 percent of the drugs sold, they could enforce such a system. They pay our taxes and could be penalized if they do not cooperate. When we discover weak or harmful drugs, we must fine or ban overseas companies from our marketplace.

The money received must go into the general tax revenue. It should never go back to the FDA because, like user fees, this works like a kickback. This system I suggest might substitute for all the rules, checklists, investigative work, and inspectors riding around on bad roads in foreign countries. Why should we care about the manufacturing process if the ultimate results are acceptable?

CHAPTER 14

PATIENT TIPS: SURVIVAL IN DRUG WORLD

DRUG WORLD IS A SHOCKING PLACE. We must face this unpleasant reality if we do not want to surrender our health to corporate marketers. Few doctors understand and fewer admit that our system is nearly anarchy. Inside the Pharma companies, the denial is even deeper. They have hundreds of thousands of nice, well-meaning, and even idealistic people. Peter Rost explains in his book *Whistleblower* (2006) how group behavior and peer pressure transform these ordinary individuals into a criminal hive, a situation analogous to war crimes. He was an executive for several of these companies.

Can we trust any medications? A limited set are essential for healthcare. Many have addictive qualities, because our bodies try to adapt to them. These include opioids for pain, all drugs used for psychiatry, and most drugs used for neurology. Aspirin, statins, and calcium channel blockers also cause withdrawal syndromes. Even diuretics (water pills), which are harmless compared to others, may put patients who quit them through weeks of swelling.

You may now think most drugs are a net harm, and I agree. Since side effects can be serious, taking anything is a risk. Once you understand this, you may discontinue some of yours.

If you try to quit, get help from your doctor. Doing your own reading and preparation makes it easier to work with them. It will also give you the confidence to decide for yourself. You learn that some health rules you thought were rigid are actually flexible.

The first principle is to avoid drugs if you can. For example, it is all right to say no to cancer treatments that work poorly or not at all (see the *Failed Cancer Treatments* chapter later). Another example: some drugs used to control heart rhythm kill more people than they save. If you are treated with one, be sure you understand why.

Drugs prescribed solely to alter laboratory readings are mostly inadvisable. Perhaps you have been told that there is something wrong with your blood pressure, cholesterol, sugar, or bone density. For each of these, lifestyle changes have more benefits than drugs. Question every prescription.

At WorstPills.org, they "list the drugs we and our consultants think you should not use. For each of these, we recommend safer alternatives." This excellent website is worth the small yearly fee. Their simple rule is to wait seven years after drugs go on the market before using them. Lack of efficacy and harmful side effects are usually apparent by then.

They describe the "seven deadly sins" of medication use. You can often spot them, even if your physician does not. The following are from their superb article, "Misprescribing and Overprescribing of Drugs."

✪ Treating side effects of one drug with more drugs.

✪ Prescribing drugs when life-style changes are more effective.

✪ Using drugs that do not work. Virus treatment with antibiotics is an example.

✪ Use of new drugs rather than the simplest and cheapest.

✪ Prescribing multiple drugs that interact with each other.

✪ Multiple drugs are used rather than just one.

✪ Prescribing doses that are too high.

If you decide that you need medications, price-shop them. Several websites show the cheapest costs for each insurance plan. You can often find drugs for even less than your copay. See:

✪ HealthWarehouse.com

✪ GoodRx.com

✪ BlinkHealth.com

✪ WeRx.org

✪ Costco and Sam's Club

✪ Independent and grocery store pharmacies

✪ Shopping outside the US (see below)

Watch your retail pharmacy closely to avoid being over-charged. They are not like a grocery store. Price shopping for food is natural, you understand it, and in some stores, prices are nearly wholesale anyway. Since you rarely go to the pharmacy, price comparison is more difficult. You know much less about drugs than the pharmacist, and they will gouge you if you are not careful.

For example, the mupirocin antibiotic ointment (oil-based, Bactroban brand), went off patent and now costs $10 a tube. The company later patented a cream (water-based) and priced it at $80. Know the difference, or they will sell you the expensive type. The ointment is better for most things, anyway.

Generic vs patented drugs: The flip-side of price shopping is that you may be handed cheaper generics. In theory they are identical, but the quality control on foreign-manufactured generics is inferior to the brand names, and this may translate into problems for you.

Since you often get a different generic every time you re-order, you may find some are weaker or problematic in other ways. I have observed this when prescribing calcium channel blocker blood pressure medications. The patented ones seem to work better with fewer side effects. Another example: I prescribed a generic beta blocker drug called metoprolol, which was supposed to work for 24 hours. But after only 12 hours, the patient's heart rate would go up, and the patient would go into an abnormal heart rhythm called atrial fibrillation. This meant the drug was shorter acting than the manufacturers claimed. I even tried having the patient cut the pill in half and take it every 12 hours, but this worked poorly also.

Here is how drug names work: the industry usually creates both a confusing chemical name and also a catchy trade name to use when harassing doctors and patients. Celebrex, for example, has a chemical name of celecoxib. Medical journals traditionally use the chemical name. I have used whatever seems more readable here.

Since patented medications are more dependable than generics, look for them overseas. Most manufacturers sell their patented drugs in other countries at a fraction of the US price, often using another brand name. You can purchase them by mail-order from foreign pharmacies' websites. Some are over-the-counter there, making this easy.

Best of all, the prices are cheaper elsewhere. Sometimes they are 50 to even 98 percent less than in the US. In late 2017, brand name Viagra was $65 here for a single 100 mg tablet and $30 for the authorized generic. By early 2020, GoodRx.com, which compares US-based pharmacies, was offering this generic for around $12. Check for updates on their website. But various Indian websites sell the same medication for $1. I have a close friend who tried the Indian version and he said it was a little weak but worked fine.

The industry calls this reimportation, and they aggressively oppose it, supposedly to protect drug quality. Several state governments have championed their citizens' rights to order abroad, however. There were congressional fights in the early 2000s to make this lawful nationwide, but our bought-and-paid-for legislature continues to block it. The compromise seems be to leave it illegal but to not prosecute anyone.

Since the FDA does not reach out of the US, there are more quality issues abroad. A maker might fake a brand name. A generic might have no active ingredients or even contain contaminants. But by 2014, wholesalers were importing 80 percent of the drugs and ingredients used here, anyway. European pharmacies get most of their drugs from other countries as well.

PharmacyChecker.com can tell you if the medications ordered overseas are likely OK. The best policy is always *caveat emptor*. Learn as much as you can before you buy and observe the effects of anything you take. And be just as careful at Walgreens as when buying internationally.

For another point of view, scan the World Health Organization (WHO) "Model List of Essential Medicines." These are 460 mostly sensible drugs, the vast majority old generics. Dull as it sounds, it is interesting reading for most practicing physicians.

To get a flavor for this list, the only statin drug is Zocor, which has been off patent since 2006. Blood pressure medications include diuretics (water pills), a few ACE inhibitors, and some venerable off-patent calcium channel blockers. The only antidepressants are amitriptyline and Prozac, the oldest one in each category, and the only antipsychotic is another senior citizen, Haldol. They include no atypical antipsychotics. Zofran, the anti-nausea drug, somehow made the list. Levothyroxine is the only thyroid replacement recommended.

For a final perspective, I asked Ms. Google. I typed "prescription medications that work the best" on 5/22/20. This is what I saw:

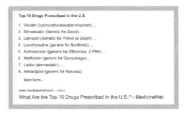

These are sensible, but at least half are phenomenally overprescribed. These include Vicodin, the two statins, and the heavily marketed antibiotic Zithromax. WHO does not recommend Vicodin (hydrocodone/Tylenol), but instead its older relative, codeine. Thyroid disease has been treated with pork thyroid since the 1890s. This is superior to levothyroxine and far cheaper. It is a complex story about how money ruins science. If you are interested, especially if you take thyroid, see stopthethyroidmadness.com or wait for publication of my book about hormones.

On the same search, down the page, Google treats us to the top earners.

These are exotics—specialty drugs, mostly for specialty diseases, with special price tags and equally special names. They treat multiple myeloma, blood clots, cancers, and inflammatory diseases. Humira, the biggest earner for two years, treats rheumatoid and other kinds of arthritis. Patients who use it may enjoy a copay assistance program, which magically transforms a bill of over $6000 a month to $35, shifting the costs onto the other insureds or the taxpayers.

Google never did tell me which drugs work the best.

PART III

LIVING ON PLANET PSYCH

CHAPTER 15

INTRODUCTION TO THE PLANET

MOST PHYSICIANS VIEW psychiatrists as somewhat feral animals. We suspect—with some justification—that many of their ideas are hot air. Unlike any other specialty, psychiatrists take care of people with normal labs and radiologic tests. They keep only patients with purely subjective problems. Psychiatrists pass patients with "organic" issues such as thyroid disease to others. These are the ones with identifiable physical signs, symptoms, and tests. Likewise, psychiatrists base treatment outcomes solely on their theories and observing patient behavior rather than on measurable, objective results.

No other specialty has a sizable group of protesters who oppose their legitimacy. These include not only Scientologists, but psychologists, scientists, journalists, and a few renegade psychiatrists. These "psychiatry deniers" believe that most psychiatric drugs used today are harmful, ineffective, and vastly overprescribed. They question the specialty's power to lock people up and force them to take damaging medications based only on their opinions.

Most of the public, however, sees psychiatry as valid,

sensible, and scientifically based. Patients expect health insurance to pay for it.

Mainstream psychiatrists believe the three primary drug categories they use—the stimulants, the SSRIs (Selective Serotonin Re-uptake Inhibitors), and the antipsychotics—are effective, beneficial, and cause little harm. Citing their close-range experience treating mental illness, they claim that these diseases are under-treated and that even patients with mild symptoms should take medications. Their studies and standards support this. But these are so structurally compromised and biased with industry money that they are useless.

These three classes of "psychoactive" medications influence sleep, wakefulness, mood, behavior, and so forth. Unlike most drugs, they enter the brain by crossing the blood–brain barrier, which is a natural microscopic defense against toxins. Drugs that behave like this can alter or damage the entire central nervous system. Although these medications are commonly used and casually prescribed, taking them is a trap because addiction is common and frequently irreversible.

As you read the next few chapters, contemplate:

1) Mental health is America's most expensive medical sector, estimated to be $213 billion in 2018 (cardiology and cardiac surgery combined might be in second place, at $143 billion).

2) A 2016 *Scientific American* source said one in six US citizens takes psychiatric medication. The Wall Street Journal said this is one in five, and the Centers for Disease Control (CDC) claims that one in four of us have a mental illness.

3) Thirteen percent of all US citizens age twelve and over received an antidepressant in 2017.

4) In the US, 9.4 percent of our children get diagnosed with hyperactivity (CDC, 2019) and about half get medication (*NY Times*, 2013).

5) Antipsychotics are considerably overused for nursing

home residents. The vast majority of demented patients get them, mainly for the convenience of the caregivers and to economically decrease staffing levels.

CHAPTER 16

"PSYCHIATRY IS IN DEEP CRISIS"

Psychiatry is the drug industry's paradise, as definitions of psychiatric disorders are vague and easy to manipulate. Leading psychiatrists are... at high risk of corruption and, indeed, psychiatrists collect more money from drug makers than doctors in any other specialty. Those who take the most money tend to prescribe antipsychotics to children most often. Psychiatrists are also "educated" with industry's hospitality more often than any other specialty. This has dire consequences for the patients.

— PETER GØTZSCHE, *DEADLY MEDICINES AND ORGANIZED CRIME* (2013)

HOW MODERN PSYCHIATRY DEVELOPED: A few decades ago, psychiatrists were losing their status. Then, the fabrication of new diagnoses along with the invention of medications to treat them saved them economically. First the antidepressants, and then the newer antipsychotics came to the rescue. This moved the specialty into the medical mainstream because the psychiatrists were the only ones who purportedly understood it all.

The novel diagnoses—some say concoctions—were enshrined in the psychiatric manual, the *Diagnostic and Statistical Manual of Mental Disorders (DSM)*. Pharmaceutical companies played a huge role in its creation.

The American Psychiatric Association (APA) started aggressive disease-mongering of the new ailments. They hired ad agencies to produce "public service" drug advertising. The corporations marketed the new supposed cures alongside.

By 2008, twenty-eight percent of the APA's income came from drug companies. According to influence theory, this made the APA virtually a subsidiary of the companies. Senator Chuck Grassley (R, Iowa) publicized the story in a congressional investigation.

Ben Furman, MD, a psychiatrist in Finland, explained how it happened in a 2018 blog:

> **The psychoanalytic belief system was thrown out and replaced with the DSM and the biomedical doctrine**: everyone should have a diagnosis, and everyone should have medication. The psychiatrists now treated all the conditions that had been treated with therapy with medication. This became the treatment of choice for almost all mental health conditions regardless of whether the patient was an adult, teenager or child. A patient without medication became a rarity. The data system of mental health services required clinicians to diagnose anyone who sought help.

The psychiatrists and corporations ignored studies showing damage from long-term drug use. They left disparaging critics out of the debate and out of the textbooks.

Finally, long after the science matured, a few of the doctors are telling the truth. In 2012, an editorial in the *British Journal of Psychiatry* said the psychiatric medication revolution was at an end. Others now echo this sentiment.

The *DSM* is a kind of chaotic bible used to promote mental diseases. With its code numbers used for insurance, some call it the billing bible. Created primarily by psychiatrists on industry payroll, it mutates and metastasizes every few years through a vote of the APA members. In 2017, after many editions, it was 947 pages long.

Insiders have decried its intellectual disarray for decades. It has become the perverse standard in the service of drug marketing. The following are a few inside opinions about it:

There was very little systematic research, and much of the research that existed was really a hodgepodge—scattered, inconsistent, and ambiguous. I think the majority of us recognized that the amount of good, solid science upon which we were making our decisions was pretty modest.

— CHRISTOPHER LANE IN *SHYNESS: HOW NORMAL BEHAVIOR BECAME A SICKNESS* (2007), QUOTING ONE OF THE *DSM*'S CONTRIBUTORS.

I pictured all these normal-enough people being captured in DSM-5's excessively wide diagnostic net, and I worried that many would be exposed to unnecessary medicine with possibly dangerous side effects. The drug companies would be licking their chops figuring out how best to exploit the inviting new targets for their well-practiced disease mongering. I was keenly alive to the risks because of painful firsthand experience—despite our efforts to tame excessive diagnostic exuberance, DSM-IV had since been misused to blow up the diagnostic bubble.

— ALLEN FRANCES, LEAD PSYCHIATRIST, *DSM IV,* AUTHOR, *SAVING NORMAL (2013)*

The National Institute of Mental Health (NIMH) in 2013 finally tossed the DSM—psychiatry's diagnostic system—into the wastebasket.

Bruce E. Levine, psychologist and journalist.

Of the 170 contributors to the most recent edition of the ...

DSM... ninety-five had financial ties to drug companies,
including all of the contributors to the sections on mood disorders
and schizophrenia... Not only did the DSM become the bible of
psychiatry, but like the real Bible, it depended a lot on something
akin to revelation. There are no citations of scientific studies to
support its decisions. That is an astonishing omission.

— MARCIA ANGELL (2011), FORMER EDITOR-IN-CHIEF OF
NEJM

The *DSM's* diagnostic categories *lack validity*, and the
NIMH will be re-orienting its research away from DSM *categories.*

— FORMER NIMH DIRECTOR THOMAS INSEL

The authors of the DSM seem more preoccupied with
politically correct jargon than substance. There are hundreds
of psychiatry blogs where participants argue obsessively
about the terminology, and there is a massive effort in each
edition to update it. For example:

They changed *Mental Retardation* to *Intellectual Disability*.
In 2010, this change was written into federal law.

Multiple Personality Disorder morphed into *Dissociative
Identity Disorder* for the DSM-V.

Other diagnoses were hatched, for example *Disruptive
Mood Dysregulation Disorder* and *Premenstrual Dysphoric
Disorder*. This was formerly *Late Luteal Phase Dysphoric
Disorder*. For many more samples, scan the entire document
online. I read it for hours and did not think it got any
better.

To understand the *DSM V* better, scan the following
excerpt:

Criteria for Oppositional Defiant Disorder:
*A pattern of angry/irritable mood, argumentative/defiant
behavior, or vindictiveness lasting at least 6 months as evidenced by
at least four symptoms from any of the following categories, and*

*exhibited during interaction with at least one individual who is not
a sibling.*

Angry/Irritable Mood:

1. Often loses temper.

2. Is often touchy or easily annoyed.

3, Is often angry and resentful.

Argumentative/Defiant Behavior:

*4. Often argues with authority figures or, for children and
adolescents, with adults.*

*5. Often actively defies or refuses to comply with requests from
authority figures or with rules.*

6. Often deliberately annoys others.

7. Often blames others for his or her mistakes or misbehavior.

Parents of boys need no other commentary unless they
support using medications with pernicious side effects to
suppress normal, but somewhat irritating behavior.

The *DSM* has worldwide influence. It is the ultimate
resource for courts, doctors, prisons, hospitals, and insurance
companies. These diagnoses lock people into legal and therapeutic boxes, but they are of dubious benefit since the drugs
work poorly and promote chronicity. Since withdrawal from
these medicines is severe and mimics the conditions treated,
long-term use becomes almost inevitable.

**The corporations blatantly falsify research to get
psychiatric drugs approved.** The study deceits I reviewed in
the FDA chapter are all used. Studies that show drugs do
not work get concealed. Positive reviews get published
multiple times, and the journals mostly only print the data
that show the drugs work. These last two tricks are such
standard practice that the drugmakers have internal nick-
names for them: "salami-slicing" and "cherry-picking,"
respectively.

Another often-used fraud is to compare massive doses of
an old drug such as Thorazine with standard doses of a new

medication. This makes the side effects of the new one look modest.

In proper drug studies, patients who take a placebo are compared with those consuming the genuine thing. However, in some psychiatric research, the people chosen to receive the sugar pill recently discontinued an older antipsychotic such as Thorazine. They are having withdrawal effects such as severe restlessness (akathisia) and anxiety. Placebo patients should not have any reactions. When such a trial is over, the lie is told that the treatment group using the drug had fewer ill effects—fewer side effects—than the sugar-pill group, which is absurd.

Psychiatric drugs are disasters. For example, Hengartner and his colleagues did a 30-year prospective study of 591 depressed Swiss adults at the University of Zurich. They found that *no* use of SSRIs (Prozac-class medications) had better patient outcomes than *some* use, which in turn had better results than *long-term* use. After nine years, they reported that the SSRIs cause more depression rather than less.

The benzodiazepines (Valium-class drugs) relieve anxiety for a few weeks. But after about a month, they stop working. After this, patients require higher dosages to produce the same effects. Later, if the drugs are discontinued, months of agonizing dread, sleeplessness, and crippling nervousness commonly occur.

The original studies of Xanax for anxiety were for 14 weeks; after four weeks, it was working; after eight weeks, it was not; and at the end of the study, as the experimenters withdrew the drug from the patients, they got much worse.

The psychiatrists and the drugmaker ignored the longer-term results and claimed there was a net benefit based on the first four weeks. (See Robert Whitaker's YouTube.) The FDA approved the drug, and it became not only the most commonly prescribed benzodiazepine but the most frequently prescribed psychiatric medication. But Xanax is addictive, and most physicians are well aware of it by now.

Other benzodiazepines are also hard to stop. Klonopin (clonazepam) is a chemically similar drug. One patient I worked with had used this 17-hour benzodiazepine to sleep every night for a decade. He decided to stop it. I wrote a compounding pharmacy prescription for smaller and smaller doses, so he tapered it over three months. He suffered with anxiety and sleeplessness the whole time, but felt better at the end. He said his energy and creativity both improved.

Another example: bipolar patients' outcomes are profoundly worse in today's medication era than they were before. Prior to the drugs, the disease often went away on its own. But now, we treat children who have psychological ups and downs with a stimulant or antidepressant before their first severe mania develops. The ones treated with antidepressants have four times increased chances of becoming "rapid cyclers," which means they have frequent recurrences.

Robert Whitaker, a distinguished journalist, summarized the horrific medication problems in *Anatomy of an Epidemic* (2010):

> *Given what the scientific literature revealed about the long-term outcomes of medicated schizophrenia, anxiety, and depression, it stood to reason that the drug cocktails used to treat bipolar illness were unlikely to produce good long-term results. The increased chronicity, the functional decline, the cognitive impairment, and the physical illness—these are usual in people treated with a cocktail that often includes an antidepressant, an antipsychotic, a mood stabilizer, a benzodiazepine, and perhaps a stimulant, too. This was a medical train wreck...*

Whitaker learned that most patients in emerging countries could not afford psychiatric drugs. Doctors there may even leave psychotic people unmedicated. The result is much less chronicity and some spontaneous cures. Almost half of the people with schizophrenia recover if they never get antipsychotics, but in the US, with treatment, this happens rarely or possibly never. History is also encouraging: before the drugs were developed, some studies showed the same thing. But since Americans now medicate practically everyone, comparison with placebo has become impossible.

In the US, mental illness, disability, and drug prescribing rose in tandem. Our psychiatric disability percentages have grown over tenfold during the modern medication era. Whittaker built a cautiously stated and well-referenced case that the medications were the cause. He also reported studies showing that within a few years, antipsychotics caused brain shrinkage in both monkeys and humans.

Psychiatrists have pressures to pass out medications. I interviewed one who said, "We cannot support our families unless we see a patient every ten minutes and give them the latest drug. Most of us know these are unproven, ineffective, and sometimes harmful, but people will not pay us just to talk with them anymore."

David Healy further describes this circus in *Pharmageddon (2012)*. The industry's interest in funding psychiatry picked up when Prozac became available in 1987. As these SSRIs and other inventions became lucrative, corporations spared no expense for psychiatrists. They cater food, pay for meetings, arrange free hotel rooms, and sometimes provide first-class plane tickets for them. Lectures, trinkets, social events, limousine service, and massive exhibit halls are all available courtesy of the drugmakers.

These companies give some working psychiatrists $300,000-$400,000 per year. This creates the desired effect; for example, one group from the American College of Neuro-psycho-pharmacology published a claim (2004) that SSRIs did not cause youth suicides. They were discredited after the discovery that nine of the ten doctors on the panel had a financial relationship with the industry.

The psychiatrists have credible excuses. The phenomena they treat are chronic and poorly understood. No labs, physical testing, or examination findings help make the diagnosis. Studying treatment is difficult because every detail is subjective. I felt sorry for them until I read about their misbehavior.

Since nothing seems to help, in their frustration, they have historically tried about anything. Ice-water baths. Electrical brain shocks—electroconvulsive therapy (ECT). Overdosing with insulin to crash the blood sugar. Even a destructive brain surgery called lobotomy, for which the inventor received the 1949 Nobel prize in medicine. These were all discredited. ECT, for example, is no longer believed to be effective and at least a third of treated patients suffer substantial memory loss. Worse, the fatality rate is 1/1000.

Psychiatrists customarily use medication combinations. They prescribe Topamax and Lamictal, which are unpleasant anti-seizure medications, to treat various symptoms and side effects. Depression, drug abuse, anxiety, and bipolar disease are all treated off-label using these. Military psychiatrists are fond of giving these seizure treatment drugs to combat troops. They often throw antipsychotics into these "drug cocktails." The side effects of all these medications include fever, hair loss, nausea, mood changes, dizziness, diarrhea, double vision, loss of appetite, and suicide.

Brexanolone is a steroid hormone approved in 2019 for postpartum depression. It requires sixty (60) hours of medically supervised intravenous injection costing $34,000.

Progesterone, a female hormone that rises during pregnancy and goes nearly to zero postpartum, can ease these symptoms. The 100 mg dose is a patent drug, but compounding pharmacies can inexpensively provide the larger doses required for this condition. There is little interest in this because there is no huge price tag.

Hallucinogens such as ketamine (which is used for date-rape) or LSD are recurrent fashions in psychiatry. Recent trials are underway to treat depression, anxiety, and post-traumatic stress disorder using small doses of these, and there is a lot of enthusiasm in some circles. LSD has been considered disreputable and classified Schedule I since the war on drugs in the 1970s, even though it has no fatal dose and its toxicities are modest compared with many prescriptions. Although these therapeutic uses may have merit, I fear they are further abuses, even though there is no patented way to profit from these older drugs—yet.

The mental health industry's ambition—now mostly realized—is to be the universal solution for every problem, and to use the drugs for nearly anyone. The National Institute of Mental Health says one in five US citizens "live with a mental illness." *Wikipedia* (2020) noted that: "Worldwide, more than one in three people in most countries report sufficient criteria for at least one [psychiatric disorder] at some point in their life. In the United States, 46% qualify for a mental illness at some point."

They were citing (respectively) the *Bulletin of the World Health Organization* and a 2005 paper by Ronald Kessler in *Archives of General Psychiatry*. He is the most widely cited psychiatric researcher in the world. He said in his paper: "Interventions aimed at prevention or early treatment need to focus on youth."

Industry financing pushes this narrative. The money passes back and forth, and it is hard to tell what is industry propaganda and what comes from legitimate psychiatric sources—if there is such a thing. For example, *MentalHealthfirstaid.org* (accessed in 2019) is a link-farm for dozens of psychiatric groups of all genders and species. It says: "In the United States, almost half of adults (46.4 percent) will experience a mental illness during their lifetime. Half of all mental disorders begin by age 14 and three-quarters by age 24."

They emphasize that besides fifty percent of adults, children, who are traditionally off-limits, should be drug candidates as well. The following chapters explain how seventeen percent of the entire US populace came to be using psychiatric drugs.

CHAPTER 17
PROZAC AND RELATIVES

The medical profession is being bought by the pharmaceutical industry, not only in terms of the practice of medicine, but also in terms of teaching and research. The academic institutions of this country are allowing themselves to be the paid agents of the pharmaceutical industry.

— Arnold Relman, MD, former editor *NEJM*
(2002)

I wrote about a thousand SSRI prescriptions over my career, which might have been a half-million dollars in drug sales. I screened my patients, as I was trained, by merely asking them a few questions.

Peter Kramer's bestselling *Listening to Prozac* (1997) duped me. He said Prozac could save patients from common symptoms of guilt, fatigue, sadness, sleep disturbance, and even aches or digestive problems. He also claimed it could be a lifestyle drug similar to today's Viagra, boosting ordinary peoples' performance. I learned later that the SSRIs are toxic, have limited utility, and the hype has produced vast overuse.

Industry marketed SSRIs as an improvement on the older

tricyclic antidepressants. These cause sedation, and only a month's supply is needed for suicide. Part of the promotion of the Prozac-class drugs was that sleepiness is mild and even enormous doses rarely cause fatality.

Before the drug era, doctors thought depression was rare and most often self-limited to about three months. Now (2020), *Wikipedia* claims that 17 percent of the US population becomes depressed during their lifetime, making them all candidates for expensive, indefinite medication usage. Legions of paid Wiki contributors, many of whom work for pharmaceutical companies, make this source only a little better than a drug industry link-farm.

A simple checklist is used to diagnose depression. A primary care medical assistant often administrates it. It is a list of nonspecific symptoms from the *DSM*. Many are opposites.

DSM criteria for depression:

✪ Depressed mood most of the time

✪ Lack of pleasure most of the time

✪ Significant weight loss or gain, appetite up or down

✪ Slow or speeded up thoughts and movements

✪ Feeling worthless or guilty most of the time

✪ Either fatigue or excess energy

✪ Cannot think or concentrate most of the time

✪ Thinking of death or suicide with or without a plan

No physical tests exist to verify the diagnosis. After waiting two weeks, doctors might commit a patient to these drugs for years—or even a lifetime. The industry promotes the disease, the medications, and the casual approach to treatment together.

"Prozac is not addictive," according to the package label written by the manufacturer. True, there are no opioid-type withdrawals. However, after discontinuation, severe anxiety and depression are common. Other issues include suicide, feeling "electric shocks," and tardive dyskinesia (TD), which is often manifest by continuous mouth movements. The drug companies claim most of this is because of the depressed state itself, rather than medication effects. There were many consumer complaints to the Federal Trade Commission about these claims that antidepressants were not addictive.

When my patients sometimes stopped the SSRI drugs and had symptoms of depression and anxiety, I believed that it was their disease and not the drug withdrawal. I was told that they must use the medications long term for them to work, so I told everyone to continue. It was bogus information, however.

The Selective Serotonin Re-uptake Inhibitor (SSRI) name was pseudoscience made up in the marketing department of SmithKline Beecham. The "chemical imbalance in the brain" idea was the brainstorm of a sales copywriter in the 1950s. Knowledge of serotonin and other neurotransmitters was even more sketchy when Prozac was invented than it is now. Today, this seductive but mythical gibberish embarrasses researchers.

Similarly, "ACE inhibitor" or "angiotensin-converting enzyme" blood pressure medications were gobbledegook names used for branding. Lithium is an old therapy for bipolar illness with no sparkling, pseudo-scientific story associated with it. It is not patented and not a money-maker, so no-one will pay a copywriter to invent a marketing idea for it. Note: lithium causes sedation and occasional tardive dyskinesia. It becomes toxic in doses only slightly higher than the therapeutic ones. This can cause permanent brain damage.

The marketers said depression was like diabetes, and SSRIs were an "insulin" for brain disease. However, no clear relationship of depression to serotonin or other neurotransmitters was ever established, and the drugs all work about the same, with a similar lack of benefit. Jill Moncrieff in The Bitterest Pills (2013) confirmed this:

No chemical imbalance or other biological process that might
explain drug action in a disease-centered way has been
substantiated for any psychiatric disorder ... Most authorities now
admit that there is no evidence that depression is associated with
abnormalities of serotonin or noradrenaline, as used to be believed
(Dubovsky et al., 2001). There is also little empirical support for the
dopamine hypothesis of schizophrenia.

Ronald Pies, editor-in-chief emeritus of the Psychiatric Times, agreed: "The 'chemical imbalance' notion was always a kind of urban legend—never a theory seriously propounded by well-informed psychiatrists... [it was a] myth."

Despite this consensus, nearly everyone still believes the metaphor and parrots the message. The idea is 1) your brain is damaged, 2) the drugs fix something, and 3) you need to take medications indefinitely.

SSRIs cause substantial harm. A 2017 literature review of randomized controlled trials in *Frontiers in Psychiatry* said these drugs are ineffective and damaging. It linked them to osteoporosis and movement disorders, including akathisia and tardive dyskinesia. They may double the risks of miscarriage and congenital disabilities. But physicians use them off label for pregnant women and during breastfeeding. Expectant mothers get severe withdrawal symptoms just like anyone else.

Sexual side effects occur in a range from 2% to 59% in various trials. In some studies, they never asked the patients about the issue. When used for premature ejaculation, about a third of men permanently improved, sometimes after just a few pills or even a single dose. This suggests significant long-terms effects that are adverse for most people. Many patients report having long-lasting problems with having orgasms after taking and then stopping these drugs.

In the first nine years of Prozac's use, between 1988 and

1996, there were 39,000 FDA complaints, a record for any drug. This included reports of suicide, psychosis, abnormal thinking, and sexual dysfunction. Many patients taking the medication have sexual difficulties, are "emotionally numb," and have "reduced positive feelings." In October 2004, the FDA introduced a written warning about suicide in children and adolescents treated with SSRIs. The agency extended this in 2006 to include young adults up to age 25.

Antidepressants are touted as *preventing* depression for people having medical problems. Prophylaxis is a market for nearly anyone.

Industry hid SSRI-related suicides and violence. The manufacturers have always claimed suicide was because of the underlying depression and not the drugs. They altogether avoided addressing violence, and the psychiatrists parroted this. Even Dr. Healy believed it before he worked as a plaintiff's expert in the Stewart Dolin case. So did I. Healy changed his mind after he read the secret corporate documents produced by the defendant corporation during the lawsuit's discovery process.

Dr. Healy learned from his review that Lilly concealed suicides. Their executives had written internally that they could "go down the tubes if we lose Prozac," and that a single big news story could do it. In 1985, a Lilly internal memorandum said that the increased suicides were 5.6 times greater than those associated with imipramine, an older antidepressant. Gøtzsche later evaluated a 2006 FDA meta-analysis of 100,000 patients and estimated that it under-reported suicide by a factor of fifteen.

SSRIstories.org has thousands of news clips about SSRI violence. Martha Rosenberg summarizes:

> *The only thing more shocking than the number of newspaper stories on the site is the number of previously healthy people who committed violence with no precipitating events. Twenty*

people mentioned here set themselves on fire. Ten bit their victims
(including a biter who was sleepwalking, and a woman on Prozac
who bit her eighty-seven-year-old mother into critical condition).
Three men in their seventies and eighties attacked their wives with
hammers. In Midwest City, Oklahoma, a woman accepted a cup of
tea from an elderly nurse she'd just met—and then strangled her. A
twelve-year-old boy left in his cousin's car while she shopped at
Target killed her five-week-old daughter, who had also been left in
the vehicle. All were under the influence of psychoactive drugs. Did
events like these ever happen before the psychoactive drug
revolution? In one month of reports on the site, a fifty-four-year-old
respiratory patient with a breathing tube and an oxygen tank and
no previous criminal record held up a bank in Mobile. An enraged
man in Australia chased his mailman and threatened to cut his
throat... for bringing him junk mail. A fifty-eight-year-old Amarillo
man with no criminal history tried to abduct three people and killed
an Oklahoma grandmother in the process. A sixty-year-old
grandmother in Seattle killed three family members and herself.
And fourteen parents drowned their children, a crime no one had
heard of before...

Lilly's publicity machine tried to claim that Scientologists perpetrated the entire story. They are well-known to hate psychiatry and their reputation is cultish, litigious, and generally unpopular.

The internal documents obtained at discovery when Lilly was sued revealed that their policy was to settle and seal Prozac cases. By 2000, they had spent about $50 million on these settlements. Other internal records showed that the corporate employees believed this was a "relatively insignificant" cost. If a lawsuit forced them to alter the labeling or withdraw the drug, losses might have been in the billions of dollars.

Completed suicides are ordinarily 4:1 men to women, but SSRI-related suicides are about the same rate for each sex. A

New Zealand study of 1829 people taking SSRIs found suicidal thinking in 39 percent. Healy did a simple one-month project where he gave Prozac to twenty healthy volunteers who had no depression. Two of the twenty had severe suicidal thoughts that slowly went away after stopping the drug. When mild depressives are treated, the primary drug effect could be akathisia, the unbearable agitation. This is the symptom Stewart Dolan experienced.

Suicides for people between 15 and 64 years old increased by a third during the era when SSRI prescribing took off. The data is from the CDC's National Center for Health Statistics between 1999 to 2017.

In *Let Them Eat Prozac* (2004), David Healy says that we are trusting the pharmaceutical companies just like patients trusted Harold Shipman, a physician who murdered over 200 people using heroin. Healy says that relationships of trust like this make serial killings easy, comparing the drug companies to killers[1].

———

PROZAC AND RELATIVES CONCLUSION

The Japanese judge antidepressants as harshly as they judge the stimulants, if that is possible. Their public health system is at least as good as ours. Taking these drugs into Japan is illegal. You can go to jail if their customs agents find Prozac in your luggage. To avoid this, you must petition them to bring your supply in with you.

Japanese studies of the SSRIs versus the older antidepressants found negligible difference, just like the Western studies. They have allowed only a few drugs of this type into their country.

German regulators did not believe Prozac was worthwhile at first. Their FDA-type agency looked at the evidence during its original approval process. They said, "Considering the benefit and the risk, we think [this drug is] totally unsuitable for the treatment of depression." They noted the patients' self-ratings in the studies showed the drug did not work. This was contrary to those of the doctors,' whose evaluations claimed it did[2]. Germany later capitulated to the drug companies and allowed Prozac into their country. However, they required a stern warning on the product labeling about issues in the first weeks of therapy and the potential need for accompanying sedatives.

Summary: SSRIs may help for severe depression, but only for a brief time. If your depression puts you in bed full time for months and you can barely resist killing yourself, you may want to risk the drugs. If you do, you must accept the risk that the medications themselves will enable you to get up and commit suicide or harm others. For moderate depression, the drugs work poorly or not at all. For mild depression, which is their current primary use, these medications are ineffective.

Casual prescription of SSRIs is unconscionable. Allowing the pharmaceutical publicity machine to promote them for brief adjustment disorders, mild sleep problems, and even grief reactions is a travesty. I wish I could say that awareness of this situation has percolated through the psychiatrists and primary care physicians. Unfortunately, industry propaganda has overwhelmed all the other narratives. In some years, SSRIs have been the most prescribed drugs, even ahead of blood pressure medications. Between 1996 and 2005, US antidepressant usage rose from 5.8 percent to 10 percent of the population, and by 2017, it was 12.7 percent.

CHAPTER 18

ANTIPSYCHOTICS ARE DISASTROUS

The person who takes medicine must recover twice, once from the disease and once from the medicine.

— WILLIAM OSLER, MD

I HAD trouble believing psychiatry was such a complete mess. I had referred people for talking therapy, and it seemed beneficial. I prescribed SSRI antidepressants and benzodiazepines such as Valium many times and had convinced myself they were helpful.

I heard the story that psychiatric hospitals had emptied soon after the antipsychotics became available. My psychiatrist colleagues were utterly convinced their medicines worked. I thought it was credible.

In medical school, they assigned me to the schizophrenia floor during my psychiatry rotation. Many people there were in the throes of deep insanity. I saw quick, dramatic improvements after we gave them medications. I read the studies that showed antipsychotics improved these symptoms for at least a few weeks. My mentors taught me that these people should continue taking the medications lifelong.

Later in my career, I treated violent and aggressive people with Haldol and Thorazine when working in the emergency department. They improved—or at least went to sleep.

I often saw patients whose symptoms recurred after stopping their medicines. When they were put back on the drugs, they mostly got better. I thought at the time that this proved the drugs worked, but I was wrong. Psychosis is commonplace during withdrawal from these addictive antipsychotic medicines.

Antipsychotic drugs work for severely impaired psychotic patients over the brief term. These people, who are often labeled schizophrenic, have a partial or complete loss of contact with reality combined with irrational or spurious thoughts, and they may hear voices. Note that visual hallucinations are something different, and usually due to drug abuse.

Patients like this are often inconvenient or intrusive for other people. They can rarely work, and a few are violent. About sixty percent attempt suicide, and fifteen percent are successful.

Antipsychotic drugs improve this group's behavior. More accurately, they suppress people's responses at the price of noxious, often permanent side effects. Hallucinations and suicidal thoughts seem to vanish—probably along with most other thoughts. Patients stop running away from home, but holding a job is next to impossible. Long-term institutionalization is the only other option to control them when they are symptomatic. This amounts to the same thing, for it always comes with drugs.

Tragically, we give the vast majority, perhaps 99 percent, of these toxic medications to people who have none of these severe symptoms. Most prescriptions are for "mood" disorders such as depression and a cornucopia of other issues, including even insomnia. Aggressive children get medicated frequently, even though the FDA does not approve these drugs for kids under five. Many are given to toddlers under two.

Health effects: "Typical" or first-generation antipsychotics such as Thorazine and Haldol were marketed as a treatment for insanity since the 1950s, but they have horrendous side effects. These include involuntary movements that look like Parkinson's disease. Rigid muscles with painful spasms are also common. Akathisia, an uncontrollable restlessness that occasionally results in suicide, occurs in 25 percent. The neuroleptic malignant syndrome, which is a violent elevation of body temperature, is rare but life-threatening.

Tardive dyskinesia (TD) is the best-known of these problems. Twenty to thirty percent of people taking these drugs get it, and 500,000 individuals in the US have it. Involuntary movements are characteristic. Patients' tongues and arms and legs may make strange motions. Their cheeks, jaws, and noses contort. Eyelids spasm, eyes move around, and the patients may make unintentional sounds. The psychiatrists call these "worm-tongue, fly-tongue, or rabbit-face." Caregivers may never recognize the drug(s) as the cause, and they may blame and punish patients.

TD usually occurs after six months to two years of treatment, but may happen after just a few months. When the drugs are discontinued, the syndrome often lingers, or sometimes it begins for the first time. Many patients who use these medications must continue them because this effect often gets worse without them. The brain's grey matter shrinks, which is a proof of damage. TD is also associated with premature death.

Antipsychotics destroy physical health. Stroke, seizures, weight gain, blood clots, heart attacks, pancreatitis, and heart rhythm disturbance are linked with them. There has never been a recall by the FDA, only a black-box warning.

The newer "atypical" antipsychotics include Abilify and Zyprexa, available since the 1990s. Their marketing proclaimed that they produced less TD and other related damage. Initial studies suggested that the tardive dyskinesia rate was a quarter of that for the older medications. Later trials focusing on TD revealed that there was little substantial difference between the older and newer drugs.

Like the first generation, the atypical antipsychotics cause health problems: stroke, blood clots, weight gain, heart attacks, and diabetes. They cut up to twenty years off of patients' lives, and they also shrink the brain. Eli Lilly, the developer, concealed these adverse effects, although they were known from the first trials.

The lawsuits: The *NY Times* reported (2007), "Lilly spent $1.2 billion since 2004 to settle lawsuits from 28,500 people who claimed they developed diabetes or heart problems after taking [Zyprexa]. At least 1,200 more lawsuits are still pending."

In 2009, the company settled a federal criminal indictment for $1.4 billion. The allegations were illegal marketing, including pushing the drug for children off-label. The fine was affordable because the gross revenue for Zyprexa was $4.7 billion in 2008 alone. They sold $4.6 billion in 2011 as the drug went off patent. According to a 2017 Kiplinger report, Zyprexa was then the thirteenth best-selling drug of all time.

In 2009, Pfizer settled allegations surrounding Geodon, another atypical antipsychotic, for $2.3 billion. These included paying physicians to increase prescribing for children. During this time, the FDA censured three of Pfizer's doctors for research misconduct, and they suspended two from working with the FDA. One, Richard Borison, received a fifteen-year prison sentence. He pled guilty to 36 charges of theft, false statements, and violation of the Racketeer Influenced and Corrupt Organizations Act (RICO). They ordered him to pay restitution of $4.26 million.

The studies and the commentary: Robert Whitaker, in *Psychiatry Under the influence* (2015), wrote that psychiatric studies had a fatal flaw: the sugar-pill control groups were distorted or absent. It is hard to find comparison patients in a society where everyone takes pills. The industry designed many trials to produce the desired results, manipulated them during their execution, or purposefully misinterpreted them.

Whitaker said that atypical antipsychotics were failures:

> **The hyping of these is now viewed as one of the more embarrassing episodes in psychiatry's history,** *as one government-funded study after another failed to find that they were any better than the first-generation antipsychotics. In 2005, the NIMH's CATIE Trial determined that there were "no significant differences" between the atypicals and their predecessors, and even more troubling, in this study, neither the new drugs nor the old ones could really be said to work.*

The medication advocates claimed this study favored the drugs.

A 2019 German analysis showed that, since 2011, over half of all the drugs they studied were worthless or no better than older medicines. Among these, psychiatric drugs were the least effective of all the recent ones entering their marketplace.

Two prominent psychiatrists, Peter Tyrer and Tim Kendall, wrote in the *Lancet* (2008) that the atypicals were now being exposed:

> *As a group, they are no more efficacious, do not improve specific symptoms, do not have a different side-effect profile than the first-generation antipsychotics, and are less cost-effective. The… atypicals can now be regarded as invention only, cleverly manipulated by the drug industry for marketing purposes, and only now being exposed. But how is it that for nearly two decades we have, as some have put it, been beguiled into thinking they were superior?*

— "THE SPURIOUS ADVANCE OF ANTIPSYCHOTIC DRUG
THERAPY."

Another commentary said that the increased costs and many other problems outweighed any advantages of the new medications (*Australian Prescriber*, 2004).

Marketing drove the atypical antipsychotics to incomprehensible profits. In 2014, the top eight psychiatric medications had $20 billion in sales, and of this, $7.2 billion was the new antipsychotic Abilify alone. It was also the top-selling drug in the US that year. Cochrane Reviews said it was no improvement over the other atypical medicines. *Consumer Reports* does not recommend it at all. Its retail cost that year was $30 to $40 for a single 2 mg pill—$2700 for a 90 day supply.

CASH PRICES OF ATYPICALS (GOODRX.COM): (Listed as brand names, but most have generics.)	
3/25/20 prices of:	**Average price:**
*Geodon 30 capsules, 80 mg	$287.29
*Zyprexa 30 capsules, 5 mg	$161.13
*Abilify 30 capsules, 5 mg	$677.40
*Promepar (Thorazine) 30 tablets, 25mg	$153.34
*Risperdal 30 tablets, .5 mg	$56.36
Saphris 30 tablets, 10 mg	$722.19
Invega Trinza (injection / 3 mo, Costco)	$8,036
Abilify Maintena (injection, 1 vial, Costco)	$2,252
Risperdal Consta (inj 1 vial 50mg, Costco)	$1,011
GoodRx offers much cheaper prices. (*off-patent, except for the injectable)	

Physicians force many patients to take these drugs. Atypicals are used for people with dementia and Alzheimer's disease, for example. But studies showed that for this group, they work no better than placebos, they double long-term dementia rates, and the patients die sooner.

There are few suitable ways to deal with sick psychiatric patients' behavioral problems because they are captives of their condition. Once they start, they are also drug captives — they cannot stop the medications without getting worse. We cannot let people run off and wander the streets or attack other residents at their facilities. And we consider physical restraints inhumane.

Current prescribing custom is to use heavy doses of medicines for nearly everyone in nursing homes. Few institutions have the caring, knowledgeable supervision required to select the least damaging and smallest quantity of drugs and then monitor their people. Even fewer institutions have sufficient staff to pursue a facility-based restraint model, i.e. locked doors, without using drugs. This is expensive.

Most people feel awful when they take antipsychotics. Some sleep all the time. Many discontinue them and they get frightening withdrawal symptoms. These may include unprovoked, uncontrollable rage. It becomes a vicious cycle of degeneration with more drugs, worsening conduct, and finally forced treatment with monthly injections. Patients believe the process is inhumane and despise it. With the use of drugs that create permanent damage, recovery from the initial problem is unlikely. There is no way to tell, anyway—the medications are taken indefinitely.

Studies show more suicides for patients who have more hospitalizations and take more drugs (this might not be cause-and-effect, but I think it is). People with schizophrenia who take medicines have worse functioning over the long term than those who never used drugs (again, that this might not be causal).

The homelessness crisis, which seems like such a mystery, is easily explained. The bulk of these people have been chewed up and spit out by our psychiatric system. Many are suffering permanent consequences of using the drugs.

The mental health industry is a lot like the prison system or the Hotel California of the Eagles song—it is much easier to get in than to leave. The drugs keep patients locked in place[1].

Antipsychotics **conclusion:** Psychosis is an intractable, poorly understood problem with no known cure. Since it sometimes goes away on its own, the best thing for the patient may be to do nothing—but this is neither easy nor convenient in most cases. Social rules say that those who trespass on the rights of others need control, but coerced drugging violates individual rights. Institutional observation of patients for several months during their first psychotic episode might allow management of mild cases without medication. Since drug therapy is near-universal in the US, no one knows for sure.

CONCLUSION: LIVING ON PLANET PSYCH CHAPTERS

Working psychiatrists address formidable problems, and we must respect their experience treating severely impaired patients. There is a definite place for their drugs, even the antipsychotics, but they should only be prescribed to a fraction of those who take them now. Forcing people to take medication breaks down the doctor-patient therapeutic trust. This should be reserved for the most intractable problems.

For more healthy individuals—who are victims of the universal overprescribing—the drugs cause much more harm than good. People seem to forget that life is full of challenges. Long-term use of a pill will not fix these. Even if they were side-effect free, which they are not, these drugs just put issues off.

The atypical antipsychotics, SSRI antidepressants, and stimulants have infested healthcare through a process of industry promotion, physician payoffs, and diagnosis-creep. The antipsychotics are likely the most damaging drugs ever widely used.

With the leadership of industry and their cosseted, lapdog doctors, psychiatric medications are prescribed indiscriminately to *nearly anyone entering a physician's office with a psycho-*

logical complaint. The short-term benefits of controlling crazy, violent, and antisocial behavior has been indecently extended to decades of expensive, damaging drugging for one in six US adults. Worst of all, we push the medications into the mouths of many of our treasured children under two.

———

EPILOGUE: SUICIDES IN THE AMERICAN MILITARY

These have mirrored the rise of antidepressant and antipsychotic prescribing. Frequently, psychiatrists use these drugs together, sometimes with anti-seizure medications. This supposedly reduces headaches and produces better sleep. *Military Times* says one in six soldiers—110,000 people—take psychoactive drugs.

Larium, a drug used to prevent malaria, causes psychosis, hallucinations, delusions, paranoia, aggression, and suicides. Personnel taking the drug have committed murders. We have known about this for over a decade, but it is still prescribed.

There is almost a suicide a day in the US armed forces. By itself, this is not firm evidence that these drugs cause suicide. Soldiering is a grim job with immense stresses and occasional brain trauma. But when we use these drugs in combination, as is the military pattern, no-one knows how they perform. It has never been studied.

CHAPTER 19

PATIENT TIPS: SURVIVING PLANET PSYCH

HERE ON PLANET PSYCH, the biggest obstacle is that the psychiatrists and the rest of us look at the scene the same way. The doctors think the medicines work because they watch their patients. The rest of us all know someone (maybe us) who swears these drugs have helped them. All this seems irrefutable. Why is it necessary to debunk something so obvious?

To review: Much of psychiatric patient behavior is because of the drugs, and the most commonly seen symptoms are because of withdrawal. This mimics the conditions being treated. Rather than proving the medications work, these symptoms are proof of brain alteration or damage. This confuses every observer. Once patients take these drugs, most are stuck on them indefinitely, both because they are addicted and also because their caregivers sincerely believe the medications help.

Can you ever quit them? That depends. For some, the best path is to stay on the drugs. But if you have a strong internal compass and understand the medications, stopping them may be worth a try because you might feel better. Since withdrawal is unpredictable, you need your doctor to monitor you. A compounding pharmacy can make up progressively weaker pills for you to take during the months that this will take.

Stuart Shipko, MD, a California psychiatrist, thinks that although these drugs are not specific treatments for mental problems, they are the only alternatives for the sickest people. When his patients are considering therapy, he fully discloses the chances of TD and other permanent issues. He tells them that the medications are "neurotoxic" rather than saying they are addictive. Most people consulting him decide against using them.

He has decades of experience trying to get people off the drugs, and he says that quitting might be possible after short-term use. However, when patients have taken these medications for years, it is typically agonizing and may be futile. Some people deteriorate and a few become psychotic. Up to six months after stopping, a severe reaction such as chronic, unremitting restlessness may still occur. Medication tapering can take up to two and a half years.

Patients who quit should read the books by Peter Gøtzsche, Peter Breggin, Robert Whitaker, and Jill Moncrieff, plus the stories on survivingantidepressants.org. Gøtzsche's *Mental Health Survival Kit* (2020) is particularly valuable. This explains why psychiatric medications are such disasters and instructs how to discontinue them.

Psychoactive drugs are justified long-term only for people with crippling mental problems. Perhaps they are justified only for patients who are seriously disrupting the lives of others. When these medications are used, the patient must accept brain damage. Although using them may help behavior over the brief term, over time they make most problems worse. The system railroads many people into institutions and forces them to take medications. Patients need advocates, preferably relatives, who can help them. Judges automatically rule for commitment on the most trivial of grounds, and psychiatrists have little time to consider much but the convenience of everyone involved.

PART IV

DEVICES, JOURNALS, AND MATH

CHAPTER 20

DEVICE-MAKERS, PHARMA'S BROTHER

Follow the money.

— Deep Throat (Watergate)

INTRODUCTION: The device companies use the same playbook as the pharmaceutical companies. Their total sales are nearly a third of the drugmakers, their FDA oversight is scanty, and their criminal settlements are similar. Like drugs, some of their products are vital, but like the drug companies, they bring many useless products to the market every year. Often these get sold for a while before being recalled when problems are discovered. The approval process is loose.

At least ten percent of us, possibly 70 million Americans, have these appliances inside us. The top 11 devices, by the number used, are:
- ✪ eye lens implants
- ✪ ear tubes
- ✪ coronary stents
- ✪ knee replacements
- ✪ screws to repair bone fractures
- ✪ intrauterine devices (IUD)

✪ spinal fusion hardware

✪ breast implants

✪ heart pacemakers

✪ artificial hips

✪ implantable defibrillators

The most unmistakable successes include cataract lenses, pacemakers, and hip replacements. After decades of placing breast implants, my opinion is that they also change patients' lives. IUDs are an accepted birth control method. The newest types work by delivering tiny amounts of hormone.

In 1938, after drug fatalities, legislation was required before the FDA allowed medications on the US market. One or two research studies using thousands of people are now required to get a medication patent. Appliances were developed and regulated much later. When the FDA was put in charge of them, the ones manufactured earlier were "grandfathered." This means approval without formal evaluation based on a history of successful use.

More recently, the FDA approves ninety-five percent or more of new devices nearly automatically, with a rule that allows recent ones on the market that are "substantially similar" to older ones. This 510 (k) clearance allows marketing with little testing. Those few that get tested more carefully rely on studies of only tens or hundreds of people, often in a single trial. Time after time, products entering the market through this process get recalled because of patient harm. The following are stories of medical device disasters over the past few decades.

HERNIA MESH: Eleven percent of all US women have had operations for pelvic stretching. This is a significant issue. It sometimes results in internal organs coming out of the vagina. Doctors performed the procedure with stitches initially, but this does not always work. In the 1970s, gynecologists began using synthetic mesh to reinforce the area. They made claims that this decreased the chances of secondary surgery, though many studies contradicted this.

Manufacturers eventually introduced over a hundred proprietary mesh products under the permissive 510 (k) rules. They each cost about $2000 for the material used in one surgery. By 2010, at least 10,000 procedures like this were being performed annually. Severe complications occurred since the early 2000s, when these operations first became common.

The mesh sometimes caused pelvic pain, menstrual difficulties, and occasionally extruded through the vagina. Worse, since it becomes incorporated into the delicate tissues of the bladder, vagina, and other areas, it was difficult to remove surgically. Cochrane reported that the quality of the studies supporting mesh were inadequate and that any advantages it offered were likely to be theoretical.

The situation was so outrageous that the mesh makers were soon forced out of business. In 2011, after public pressure, the FDA held hearings and required studies. Of the 34 original manufacturers who were mandated to do investigations, only four began trials to examine the five remaining mesh products. In 2016, the FDA started requiring studies before licensing, and as of November 2018, only three products were still on the market awaiting approval.

In late 2018, pelvic suspension procedures using mesh were forbidden in British government hospitals. On April 16, 2019, the FDA ordered manufacturers to cease selling and distributing mesh for most gynecologic procedures. In 2020, Johnson and Johnson lost a $344 million judgment because of their false and deceptive marketing of mesh products. They could afford it: their gross revenues in 2018 were $81.6 billion.

ESSURE is a coil of metal placed in a woman's fallopian tubes for lifetime sterilization. The company made the claim that this procedure was less invasive and cheaper than laparoscopic tubal ligation. In 2002, the device was approved in the US based on two short-term studies. These began with 745 patients, but by two years, fewer than 200 women were still in the trials.

Nickel sensitivity caused allergic-type reactions for some. Ten to twenty percent of the population is well-known to be allergic to nickel. I cannot fathom how a sophisticated medical device company would cut corners like this and use cheap metal. Even costume jewelry makers know that they should not use nickel because it causes skin rashes. Other patients had pelvic pain, heavy periods, spotting during ovulation, and even perforation of the uterus or fallopian tubes. Some coils shifted to other places in the abdominal cavity. Extrusion into the vagina occurred in fully 10 percent of cases.

For removal of the device, an extensive surgery with an incision in the fallopian tubes was necessary. Some patients required hysterectomies. Gynecologists who attempted to pull the coil out through the uterus often left fragments.

The device was removed from the European market in 2017. *The Bleeding Edge,* an exposé film about women damaged by the product, was released in 2018. After this, Essure was quickly and "voluntarily" withdrawn from the US.

CARDIAC STENTS are an ingenious invention that physicians insert into a blocked area of an artery to hold it open. They are barely effective—if the risks and prodigious expenses are ignored. Cardiologists get paid thousands of dollars for each one. Some seem to place as many as they can.

Dr. Midei of Baltimore, Maryland, was a champion stent installer, putting in about 1200 a year. He had a close relationship with Abbott Laboratories, a stent maker. Along with everything else, they gave him a $2,159 roasted-pig barbecue the day he inserted a record 30 stents. A review of his work by others revealed 585 unnecessary procedures costing $6.8 million over two years. Medicare had paid over half of it. His hospital confessed they were kicking back money to him for referrals and paid a $22 million settlement. Midei lost his medical license.

The New York Times quoted Steven Nissen, chief of cardiology at the Cleveland Clinic: "What was going on in Baltimore is going on right now in every city in America… patients … have been given multiple unneeded stents. We're spending a fortune… on procedures that people don't need."

At Mount Sinai Hospital in New York, cardiologist Samin Sharma was even busier than Midei. He proudly claimed 1500 complex cardiology interventions a year that cost $2.75 million. These procedures were often $20,000 each, and his total income was $4.8 million. Sharma got his hospital to open their cardiac catheterization laboratory 24 hours a day so stents could be placed continuously. Mount Sinai went from losing more than $50 million a year to gross revenues over a billion dollars by 2006.

In 2009, Louisiana physician Mehmood Patel was sentenced to ten years in prison for inserting unnecessary stents and billing fraud.

Just what is unnecessary? With few exceptions, stents for heart disease are useless. I tell the story in a later chapter. The medical boards have not caught up with this and rarely revoke licenses for stent placement.

IMPLANTABLE VAGAL NERVE STIMULATORS were the central story of Jeanne Lenzer's book *The Danger Within Us* (2017). This nerve's function is to help control the throat muscles, influence the heart rate and the gut, and carry sensation from the internal organs. Stimulating it electrically is claimed to produce near-miraculous effects for dozens of conditions.

Lenzer reported a case where the stimulator was stopping the patient's heart at intervals. Even after doctors turned the device off, problems continued. The implant and its wires caused severe scarring in the vital areas around it, so

complete removal without damage was impossible. After
suffering these effects, the patient read the studies for the
machine and found little evidence that it worked for
anything.

However, the company recommends the device for treatment of depression, anxiety, atrial fibrillation, autism,
bulimia, burn-induced organ dysfunction, and "drop attacks"
as well as fibromyalgia, heroin-seeking behavior, hiccups,
multiple sclerosis, inflammation of the heart (myocarditis),
obesity, rheumatoid arthritis, congestive heart failure, and
ringing in the ears. Experienced physicians know a treatment
said to cure everything is likely a fraud, or to say this more
politely, a placebo.

The FDA initially refused to approve the stimulator. So the
company hired an aggressive, flamboyant venture capitalist,
Skip Cummins, to promote it. He convinced St. Jude Medical
to invest $12 million to fund a study, and this showed seizure
reduction. He persuaded the FDA to approve the device, even
though there were 17 deaths in the first 1000 patients.

By the time of Lenzer's publication, the instrument had
become FDA-approved for migraines, cluster headaches, and
depression. Doctors were soon using it off-label for dozens of
other conditions. A Senate Finance Committee investigated
the 2006 FDA approval. They found that Daniel G. Schultz,
Director of the Center for Devices and Radiology and Health,
overruled twenty FDA officials to allow the vagal stimulator
on the market. This was the first time the FDA ever approved
a device against the unanimous opposition of the internal
scientists and administrators.

Lenzer summarizes the evidence against vagal stimulator
treatment of seizures: "The... research data, stripped of the
emotional sway of anecdote and the misleading presentation
of 'significant' findings of 'benefit,' added up to this: 18
percent of test subjects improved in the short term, most
patients failed to improve, there was no—or questionable—

benefit over the long term, some patients experienced substantial worsening, and a concerning number died."

VERTEBROPLASTY is used to treat compression fractures, which are an internal crushing and shortening of one or more vertebrae. These are painful, usually spontaneous, and occur mostly in the elderly.

A Superglue-like substance, acrylic cement, is injected into the affected bony segment. Initial observational studies with small numbers gave the impression this reduced pain. Radiologists could do it, so they had a procedure that competed with the orthopedic surgeons. When insurance and Medicare started paying, it turned into an industry.

Two groups, one in America and one in Australia, performed sham comparison studies. They did the actual procedure for some patients, and in others, they did a faked invasive procedure without the injection. The trial showed no difference in either pain or disability between these groups. Cochrane also reviewed the situation (2018) and agreed that the procedure did not work.

Dr. Kallmes was one innovator in the US and had been performing vertebroplasty for fifteen years. He continued to do it even though he said the study results shocked him. Australian radiologists published rebuttals to the studies and kept performing the procedure. Other trials are ongoing. American radiologic and neurologic surgical societies recommended the continuation of insurance and Medicare reimbursement.

Australia stopped paying for vertebroplasty in 2011. America and the UK still pay for it, and it costs about $3000. Recently, radiologists invented kyphoplasty or "balloon" vertebroplasty. This involves putting a balloon into the crushed vertebrae before injecting the cement. A sham control study, "Vertebroplasty versus sham procedure for painful acute osteoporotic vertebral compression fractures," proved kyphoplasty was a failure (*BMJ*, 2018). A review of the literature, also in 2018, said it was a placebo. It costs $8000.

To restate the obvious: any decent study determines defin-itively if a procedure is effective. If there is controversy after the research is over, the method does not substantially work. Financial interests inevitably cloud judgment.

INFERIOR VENA CAVA (IVC) FILTERS were invented in the 1970s. Most blood clots or emboli of the lungs travel from leg veins, and this can be fatal. The IVC devices put a physical barrier between the leg veins and the lungs. Patients who already had emboli were candidates for them. Between 1999 and 2010, one in six Medicare patients with a history of lung emboli received an IVC filter to prevent more.

But these devices cause bleeding, more clots, and other problems. The studies on them are poor quality and do not show any improved patient survival that would justify their use. In trauma cases, the filters cause more harm than good. Ido Weinberg, assistant professor of medicine at Mass-achusetts General Hospital, summarized: "Many physicians would say that these devices are being used too often, that they are being used for the wrong indications, and that they are associated with significant harm." The American College of Chest Physicians now recommends them only for unusual circumstances, such as patients who had a pulmonary embolism who cannot use anticoagulants.

No-one has any idea about the total number of devices inside Americans. There is no registry or reporting require-ments. The only database is voluntary, the FDA's Manufac-turer and User Facility Device Experience. The only regulation so far (2014) directed device manufacturers to embed unique device identifiers (UDIs), starting with knees, cardiac valves, and artificial hips. This is like a bar code. A register will be in place by 2020, but there are no plans to inte-grate it with patients' medical records.

Jeanne Lenzer wrote, "Walmart tracks every single head of

lettuce it buys and sells and can determine how many heads of lettuce are on its shelves at any given moment, yet no one —not the FDA, not Brookings, not anyone—can say how many people are dying because of implanted medical devices. It's a black hole."

The guesses about deaths from medical devices range from 3000 to 160,000 a year (from Brookings nonprofit public policy organization and others).

Less than five percent of approved devices get formally studied, and trials are often poor quality. Many are observational, which is a study without a control group. The trials of the Essure tubal implant and the vagal nerve stimulator were like this, so it is impossible to tell whether these devices work.

Corporations who do the studies often conceal injuries and deaths as trade secrets. Lenzer believes something like this happened with the stimulator.

A Supreme Court decision (Riegel v. Medtronic, Inc., 552 US 312, 2008) protected devices from most lawsuits. It exempts the companies from litigation if the FDA agreed on the device's effectiveness and safety during the approval process. When the drugmakers have issues, they may have to defend lawsuits, but this Supreme Court decision protects the appliance manufacturers. The only protection left for the patients is that the FDA can later revoke a product's approval.

This lax oversight and minimal study requirement result in the FDA recalling 1100 devices every year. The "dogs" are seldom weeded out before approval. These recalls are serious for patients.

When medications are stopped, there are few long-term consequences except with psychiatric drugs. Devices, however, may require a hazardous surgery to take them out, and removal may be unsuccessful. With every operation to replace or remove an implant, about the same percentage dies as during the original procedure. For example, hip implant surgeries kill between 1/300 and 1/400 patients.

Steven Tower, an orthopedist, started having tremors and then a mental breakdown. He discovered his cobalt hip implant was giving him blood levels of the metal that were 100 times normal. When the device was removed and replaced, all the muscles around his hip were grey and black. They were contaminated with cobalt.

He recovered, and the experience turned him into an activist. By 2010, the company recalled the prosthesis from ninety thousand US patients.

Implantable defibrillators are designed to prevent death by shocking the heart to correct rhythm disturbances. One brand began to randomly and painfully discharge. A friend told me about this happening to him. He said it felt like a horse had kicked him and knocked him to the ground. The company recalled 300,000 of these devices between 2007 and 2011. Most of these patients had coronary heart disease, so the removal process was especially risky.

The US implantable device industry's gross revenues were more than $136 billion in 2014. The worldwide total was $300 billion, nearly a third of the pharmaceutical industry's. Profit margins are similar: 20 to sometimes 30 percent. Like the drugmakers, tax and insurance money pays them. The average CEO of the top 18 device companies made over $15 million a year in 2015.

Some authors get rich just by writing about these products. A 2013 Senate investigation found that the Medtronic device company paid $210 million to physicians who concealed adverse results in their reports. One doctor fabricated literature about a bone growth product without revealing its hazards and got $23 million.

The companies paid some spine surgeons $4000 a day for unspecified services, presumably to use the products for their patients.

These device corporations have colossal criminal and civil settlements. They can afford it, however. Medtronic, for example, had gross revenues of about $30 billion in 2018. The following is Medtronic's partial legal history, which speaks for itself.

✪ $75 million paid in 2008 to settle false claims relating to bone cement products.

✪ $23.5 million settlement in 2011 for paying money to doctors for implanting pacemakers and defibrillators.

✪ $85 million paid in 2012, settling a class-action lawsuit regarding illegal promotion of bone graft material for off-label usage.

✪ $9.9 million paid in 2014 for reimbursing doctors who implanted pacemakers and defibrillators.

✪ $2.8 million in 2015 for sales of a spinal stimulation device without FDA approval.

✪ $4.4 million in 2015 for falsely labeling devices made in the USA so they could be sold to the US military.

✪ In 2016 they admitted they failed to report over 1000 adverse events for their spinal stimulation device. No fines or penalties were imposed.

✪ Medtronic gave tens of millions of dollars to surgeons for "consulting" and other schemes to promote the use of surgical hardware. Back fusion devices cost about $13,000 per case. One doctor received $400,000 in a year for eight days of his time. Another got $700,000 over nine months.

Other device companies are similar:

✪ Johnson and Johnson (J&J) was fined $84.7 million in 2007 for kickbacks to orthopedic surgeons who were installing their knee and hip devices.

✪ J&J paid $70 million to settle criminal and civil charges of bribing overseas doctors (2011).

✪ In a 2007 plea bargain, five other manufacturers admitted paying surgeons tens to hundreds of thousands of dollars to use their hip and knee products. The fine was $311 million.

✪ Biomet paid $29 million in fines between 2012-14 for similar allegations.

Since patient-first is not the primary corporate value, issues such as I describe here are frequent. Federal prosecutors exert little control. Jesse Eisinger in *The Chickenshit Club* (2017) says the system is broken: "Defaulting to a settlement without prosecuting individuals corrodes the rule of law... (and) corporate officers possess... the ability to commit crimes with impunity. Such injustice threatens American democracy." If we had the power and the will to break up one of these corporations, we would see the behavior improve for others.

Investors may have more power than the FDA to punish corporations, but their interest is in stock prices rather than patients. For example, Medtronic's kyphoplasty procedure to correct vertebral compression fractures lost credibility. This caused the stock to crater despite all the money given to doctors. Most issues do not affect product sales, markets, or executive compensation, so the company factors the settlements into the expenses, and profits continue.

Summary: Some devices are like miracles. I had cataract surgery, and it was almost as easy as cleaning foggy lenses. All the colors were brighter after the procedure, and I threw away my distance glasses. I was awake during the process, and there was no pain. I also have screws in one knee, mesh in my inguinal hernias, and I know a lot about breast implants. Some of my friends have artificial hips, and they nearly all function without pain.

Like the rest of medicine, you must research before you consent to the use of implants. Never forget that we allow these things on the market with inadequate testing. This is an outrageous oversight that must be reformed. Newer is rarely better—it means only that the devices are unproven.

CHAPTER 21

THE JOURNALS' SINS ARE
THE EDITORS' SINS

*If you don't read the newspaper, you're uninformed. If you read the
newspaper, you're misinformed.*

— MARK TWAIN

CORPORATE FUNDING HAS MADE medical journals wealthy.
When I trained 35 years ago, they were everywhere, but with
the cash injection you will read about below, they have
become a blizzard of paper on every surface of a doctor's
house and office. To scan the primary care articles alone
would take hundreds of hours a month. Over 5,000 journal
articles get published every day.

Physicians get their information from journals, and the
editors are responsible for everything that gets printed. They
are the most sophisticated people in healthcare, and they
understand what is happening as it occurs. But they only
speak up after they retire because they do not want to lose
their prestigious, lucrative jobs (I am guilty of this, too).

The following are two of their confessionals. There are
similar statements published about *NEJM*, *JAMA*, and others.

Journals have devolved into information laundering operations for the pharmaceutical industry. The case against science is straightforward: much of the scientific literature, perhaps half, may simply be untrue. Afflicted by studies with small sample sizes, tiny effects, invalid exploratory analyses, and flagrant conflicts of interest, together with an obsession for pursuing fashionable trends of dubious importance, science has taken a turn towards darkness.

— RICHARD HORTON, *LANCET* EDITOR

Medical journals are an extension of the marketing arm of pharmaceutical companies.… between two-thirds and three-quarters of the trials published in the major journals — Annals of Internal Medicine, JAMA, Lancet, and New England Journal of Medicine — are funded by the industry.

— RICHARD SMITH, EDITOR, *BRITISH MEDICAL JOURNAL*
AND AUTHOR, *THE TROUBLE WITH MEDICAL JOURNALS*
(2006)

About half of journal revenue comes directly from drug companies. Perhaps 90 percent of the articles and research are industry-funded, and the industry's contractors ghostwrite the majority. Marcia Angell, the *NEJM* editor for 20 years, told how they do it in *The Truth About the Drug Companies* (2004), "I saw companies begin to exercise a level of control over the way research is done that was unheard of when I first came to the journal… It is simply no longer possible to believe much of the clinical research that is published, or to rely on the judgment of trusted physicians or authoritative medical guidelines."

A review of 370 drug studies in 2003 showed that industry-sponsored trials were much more likely to have positive results than when funding was from other sources. A single positive trial may be printed and reprinted in hundreds of different venues and forms. The core of science is unfavorable reports, but these are frequently concealed. For example, during the approval process for the influenza treatment Tamiflu, the drug company withheld the Australian studies that suggested the drug was worthless.

If a journal publishes something their industry sponsors dislike, they will threaten them with loss of advertising or worse. *Annals of Internal Medicine* (June 1992) made the mistake of publishing Michael Wilkes' study about drug advertising harms. The NEJM and JAMA had turned down the article.

In punishment, the big corporations withdrew advertising from the *Annals*, and they lost over a million dollars in revenue. Two respected editors lost their jobs. After this, US journals allowed pharmaceutical companies to print written rebuttals of any study they did not like in the same issue as the study. Neither big tobacco nor big food has ever received a concession like this.

Journals make startling amounts of money. Profit margins at scientific publishing companies average a sensational 35 percent. Other successful publishers worldwide average 10 percent, and industries without subsidies are successful at 10 percent. Reed Elsevier, the largest medical publisher, is stunningly profitable:

YEAR:	REVENUE:	NET:	PROFIT:
2016	3.28 b	1.22 b	37%
2010	2.58 b	933 m	36%

How do they do it? Journals' expenses are modest. Industry, federal grants, and academia pay for studies, so these are free. Review editors and members of editorial boards are mostly unpaid volunteers. Revenues are huge, however. A single journal subscription may cost several thousand dollars a year. Reprinted articles from a journal often cost $50 each. Comprehensive literature searches can cost tens of thousands of dollars to get the full texts.

Journals were billing Harvard's library $3.5 million a year

for subscriptions. It had to cut some journals from their list because of these ever-increasing costs. In 2019, the University of Southern California ended its subscription to Elsevier's journals because of the exorbitant prices.

Reprints make money for the journals because they sell them right back to the study sponsors. These companies typically pay for the entire charade, from study design to research grants to ghostwriting. Salespeople gift purchased articles to doctors to prove that the drugs work. This is a page from the corporate sales and influence playbook. Dr. Deepak Malhotra described the way it works in the *BMJ*: "As a medical director of a pharmaceutical company, I learnt how to get articles published in journals, with one journal promising publication if we purchased 2000 reprints at $10 each."

The *NEJM's* publisher gets 23% of its income from reprints. *The Lancet*—41%. *JAMA* receives 53%. In a 2012 study, reprint income per article for the *Lancet* was a median of £287,353 ($363,946), with the most profitable one £1,551,794. Industry funding was ten times more likely in the most reprinted articles. Journal volumes labeled "special editions" are advertising vehicles. They look like the others but usually describe only a single therapy, and the journal editors do not expect them to have high scientific standards. One drug company typically supplies nearly the entire budget.

Occasionally, industry fabricates entire journals, and they look legitimate. Merck created the *Australasian Journal of Bone and Joint Medicine* to advertise Fosamax. Recall the *Disease-Mongering* chapter; this drug's utility is doubtful. The Medline database did not index this journal, and it had no website. Elsevier published the magazine for several months, then it vanished.

The industry pays journal editors directly, and they get their salaries in addition. Jeanne Lenzer describes how the device companies use this power:

*A medical journal editor who received millions of dollars from a
medical device manufacturer wrote and edited articles favourable to
the manufacturer without stating his conflict of interests to readers.
Thomas Zdeblick, a University of Wisconsin orthopaedic surgeon…
editor-in-chief of the Journal of Spinal Disorders & Techniques in
2002, received more than $20m… in patent royalties, and $2m in
consulting fees from Medtronic for spinal implants sold by the
company during his tenure as editor.*

— *BMJ* (2010)

Jason Fung, a Canadian academic nephrologist, summarizes these payouts in a blog:

*Of all journal editors that could be assessed, 50.6% were on
the take. The average payment in 2014 was $27,564. Each. This
does not include an average $37,330 given for 'research'
payments… Each editor of the Journal of the American College of
Cardiology received, on average, $475,072 personally and another
$119,407 for research. With 35 editors, that's about $15 million in
money for editors. No wonder the JACC loves drugs and devices.*

Medium.com (2018)

The massive advertising revenues, the reprint deals, and
the payoffs to the editors create near-complete corporate
control of the only physician information source. We support
the drugmakers and device manufacturers with insurance
and government dollars, and they pay the journals and
editors. The "big five" most respected medical journals,
Lancet, JAMA, BMJ, NEJM, and Annals of Internal Medicine,
are all contaminated with this commercial bias. The BMJ has
the most integrity, at least by one measure. Only three percent
of its revenues come from reprints.

Business corrupts science when it pays for research.

Nortin Hadler wrote in *The Citizen Patient* (2013): "It turns out that the vast majority of the clinical literature is so lacking in methodological quality as to offer no contribution of substance to clinical decision making. For most clinical questions, one is fortunate to find a dozen studies that can be deemed informative." Gøtzsche is franker: "The pervasive scientific misconduct has led to a research literature where one has to dig deeply to find the few gems among all the garbage."

CHAPTER 22

EASY MATH EXPLAINS EVERYTHING

THIS IS AN INTERMISSION—YOU may need it by now. This chapter explains the simple math that should be used to decide if treatments work.

Nobel laureate Richard Feynman explains scientific studies: "If something is true, really so, if you continue observations and improve the effectiveness of the observations, the effects stand out more obviously." This rarely happens in medicine. Most of our studies are paid for by corporations and involve enormous numbers of patients. The groups being compared rarely show sizable differences. Physician-statisticians alter the results to satisfy whoever writes their check. This usually involves concocting "statistically significant" conclusions from tiny differences. They routinely make questionable therapies appear acceptable.

Good scientists know that proper studies of patients most often prove credible theories dead wrong. Good scientists do not get fooled by theories or plausible reasoning. *Good scientists know that all unconfirmed ideas, no matter how convincing, will likely be proven wrong—because this is what happens most of the time.*

But now, instead of dismissing therapies when studies

prove them ineffective, endless controversies arise and drugs move into production based on shreds of evidence. Expensive testing, risky therapies, and even treatments for healthy people—where harm outweighs the advantage—are promoted. It is an assembly line of fakery.

As you begin to understand the squabbling over microscopic differences in our ghostwritten medical journals, meditate about smoking. This causes one in five US deaths. A study with results as strong as this is indisputable, but this rarely happens in healthcare.

———

THE NUMBER NEEDED TO TREAT (NNT)

This is the number of individuals who need to receive a therapy for one to benefit. This typically means that one person will have a bad result prevented. To arrive at this figure, a group of people that is treated is compared with a group who is not. If one percent benefits in the treated group, the NNT is 100, for example.

The NNT is a rule of thumb. It is not typically reported in medical journals, but calculating it is a straightforward way to see whether a therapy is worthwhile. Nortin Hadler, a biostatistician, writes: "If I have to treat more than twenty patients to do something really meaningful for one, I regard the treatment as marginal." He also says an NNT of 50 "is too small a health benefit to measure reliably" and that treating 50 to produce an improvement for one is the absolute cutoff. If more are needed, Hadler says that the effects are barely measurable and probably would not happen again if studies were repeated.

Hadler reported in his 2008 book Worried Sick that the following therapies do not have an NNT of even 50, according to the best reviews available then:

✪ *Coronary artery bypass grafts, angioplasties, or stents to save lives or improve symptoms*
✪ *Arthroscopy for knee pain*
✪ *Any surgery for a backache*
✪ *Statin therapy to reduce cholesterol and thereby save lives*
✪ *Newer antidepressants for situational depression*
✪ *Drugs for decreased bone density*
✪ *PSA screening and radical prostatectomy to save lives*
✪ *Screening mammography to save lives*
✪ *Many a cancer treatment to save lives*

Other medical statisticians believe it reasonable to treat up to a hundred patients to produce one benefit. If this was true, some therapies above look more useful. Certainly, treating over a hundred patients to produce a favorable result in one patient is quackery, not medicine. Much of what we doctors do falls in this category.

The following are a few clarifications.

1) *TheNNT.com* explains this concept in more detail and summarizes hundreds of diseases with favorable and unfavorable NNTs.

2) The number needed to treat measures benefits. It does not address harms.

3) When a serious consequence such as death or heart attack is measured, more people might be reasonably subjected to a therapy to avoid it. Here, higher NNTs might possibly be justified.

———

STATISTICAL TRICKERY: RELATIVE VS ABSOLUTE RISK IN MEDICAL STUDIES

Study authors and the media often report results in terms of RELATIVE rather than ABSOLUTE numbers, which vastly overstate the advantages of a therapy. Here is how it works.

To understand this, consider a medication that cuts heart attack rates in half, from 2 percent a year to one percent. This RELATIVE risk improvement sounds great, but it is misleading and some would say fraudulent. The all-important ABSOLUTE risk improvement—decrease in heart attacks for everyone who gets the therapy—*is only one percent.* Only one percent of those who took the drug benefitted.

The characteristics of the group that receives therapy is critically important. If the patients who are treated have severe heart disease with a heart attack rate of 25 percent instead of two percent a year, cutting this in half would be consequential. The ABSOLUTE improvement is still 50 percent but the RELATIVE improvement is 12.5 percent when the 25 percent heart attack rate is cut in half.

Absolute risk reduction and the NNT are reciprocals. In the first example, 100 patients need to be treated to produce one result, an number needed to treat of 100, which is not good. In the second example of patients who have severe heart disease, the NNT is 8, a very favorable number (100/12.5).

So, when effective therapies are used to treat people with real problems, the math works. Treating or screening everyone else, on the other hand, does not. This example is a basic introduction to the numbers surrounding the cholesterol drugs.

These statin anti-cholesterol medications are expensive and sometimes toxic, with the potential to produce brain, muscle, and other damage. They occasionally kill people. But their benefits are modest.

Here are real numbers. In one study, for patients taking the drug for five years, nonfatal heart attacks decreased by only two percent, the ABSOLUTE improvement in heart attacks. The placebo group's heart attack rate was 6.5 percent. The study authors simply divided these percentages, 2%/6.5%, to get the RELATIVE reduction in heart attacks, which is nearly a third. This deception was published and promoted. The two percent ABSOLUTE figure was the true benefit.

It gets worse. The goal of treating heart disease is not primarily to reduce heart attacks, but to decrease deaths. *This trial showed no improvement in survival,* an ABSOLUTE improvement number of *zero*. This is a much "harder" or more consequential and measurable number than heart attacks. There are other questions. Were the studies faked? Is it worth putting up with medication toxicity in many patients for five years for this result? When drug fatalities are considered, is this decrease in heart attacks worth it?

Another example: colonoscopy does not work when used to check healthy people for colon cancer. Consider: between 40 and 80 years old, about 60 percent of people die, which is their ABSOLUTE risk of death from all causes. Two percent die of colon cancer between these ages, the RELATIVE risk of death from colon cancer alone.

Do colonoscopies save lives? Assume they are performed every few years, half of the colon cancers are found, we cure all of them, and the procedure is without risk. We would save one percent of the two percent who would die. The RELATIVE improvement in colon cancer survival would be 50 percent—which sounds great. However, the ABSOLUTE improvement in all-cause deaths would be 1 out of 60, less than two percent, not much. The number needed to treat (the number needed to screen in this case) would be 100.

Colonoscopies do not work this well, however. The process is expensive, uncomfortable, humiliating, and slightly risky. Most people rarely get colonoscopies because they hate them. The procedure misses a lot of cancer, and doctors cannot cure all the ones they find. A few patients have their colons punctured, a few bleed, and some die. *After decades of study with thousands of patients, there has never been a randomized controlled study that showed screening colonoscopies lower*

ABSOLUTE (all-cause) deaths. So it does not help anyone live longer.

Imagine for a moment how journal authors fool us with the routine reporting of RELATIVE rather than ABSOLUTE risk. Most physicians do not know any better. The editors do, but they look the other way and publish anyway.

People who find blood in their stools are not part of this analysis. They come to us for *symptoms* rather than for a *checkup*. For them, since their chances of having a disease are much higher, we do colon examinations and whatever else is necessary. They might have a tumor that needs surgical removal, or they might need medication for inflammatory disease, for example.

There are a few reasonable indications for doing colonoscopies at routine intervals. These include people with Crohn's disease, ulcerative colitis, and hereditary polyposis. This last is a syndrome with hundreds of polyps inside the colon. These patients all have a much higher chance of getting cancer, and if we find it early, we save lives. Those who have children, siblings, or parents with colon cancer are also at high risk. The math works for them, too.

Mammograms save *no* lives for people without symptoms or lumps. Both the NNT and relative versus absolute risk show they do not improve ABSOLUTE survival. This has been proven using studies of enormous groups of patients. Our current process, however, is to examine everyone in certain age groups every few years. This entails enormous time, energy, money, and slightly risky follow-up surgery. But the numbers do not work.

Here is why, using actual figures. If 1000 women have mammograms for ten years, six will die from breast cancer anyway. If another 1000 women have no mammograms for ten years, nine will die from breast cancer. Three are saved, a theoretical RELATIVE risk improvement of 3/9, a third, which sounds excellent. But the ABSOLUTE improvement is only 3/1000. The number needed to screen is 1000/3, or 333, far too high to be reasonable.

After hundreds of millions of mammograms, our patients are left with expense, anxiety, biopsy scars, chemotherapy, radiation exposure, and even a rare death from the surgeries and anesthesia. When a thousand of them are screened for ten years, this is 10,000 patient-years, maybe 30,000 mammograms, and a tremendous number of biopsies and other therapies.

Hundreds of slow-growing tumors get identified and, once discovered, are treated. If no patients ever had mammograms, a lot of these would go away on their own. Neither the patients nor their doctors would ever notice anything. Other women with the cancer would die from something else despite persistence of the tumor. Treatments are a net harm for both these groups.

The open secret of medical trials is that nearly all report their results as the *meaningless* RELATIVE risk, rather than the *essential* ABSOLUTE risk. To decipher this, you must usually look at the complete study rather than just the abstract. This would not reveal faked or concealed data, but sometimes the reporting is nearly intact because most doctors are easily fooled by relative risk. Data fraud is unnecessary.

If I am still confusing you, watch this YouTube video by the brilliant David Newman, MD.

———

THE FOUR HORSEMEN OF STUDY TREACHERY:

1) Studies with a cast of thousands are suspect. Huge numbers are being used to identify tiny differences, but discoveries made like this are rarely meaningful. It might turn out differently in another study, which is rarely done. The drugs in the disease-mongering chapter are examples. Many had massive trials that supposedly showed benefits. These were used to promote the drug. Careful analysis, however, reveals that none of these medications have value for patients.

Cancer studies often use enormous numbers. Dr. Hadler, in *Worried Sick* (2008) explains:

> *The literature on… [chemotherapy]… is extensive. There are multiple trials. Some are designed to recruit thousands of patients for randomization. Whenever I see a trial with thousands of subjects, I bridle… in large trials seeking tiny effects, randomization errors can never be avoided. The very fact that the Canadian and Swedish investigators [of mammographic screening for breast cancer] felt compelled to design trials with tens of thousands of subjects followed for decades says to me that the health effect they target is too tiny to measure and too small to be meaningful. I don't think such trials should ever be done.*

Hadler admits many of his peers love humongous studies, believe they mean something, and that he is in the minority. But you do not have to subscribe to Hadler's strict math to see the conflict of interests. Vulnerable patients, sometimes at the end of their lives, are being shaken down for their health-care dollars.

2) Randomized controlled trials are worthless if there are conflicts of interest, even though this structure is the gold standard for establishing medical knowledge.

Here is how it should work. Patients are recruited to take part in a trial. Each is assigned at random to one of two groups. The treatment group receives the treatment being studied. The control group receives a placebo or an older drug. Neither the patients nor the doctors are supposed to know who is in either group until the study is done. This is called blinding.

These trials are complicated, expensive, and rife with opportunities for manipulation. When industry pays for a study, the purpose is to make money. The overriding question becomes, "Can we make it look as if the drug works?" rather than "What is the truth?" They tailor each study, before it starts, to meet the goal of drug approval. This guarantees flawed results.

For example, a study might make a comparison with either another drug or a placebo. The choice depends on which they think will make their medication look the best. If there is a concern about a new drug looking bad against an old one, they prefer placebo controls.

New numbers are sometimes cooked up, and patients in different study groups may get switched from one to another after the study is complete. A second commonly used hoax is saying that findings that are not statistically significant do not even exist. But, for example, if there are more deaths in the treatment group, this must be investigated.

When industry sponsors trials, it becomes a garbage-in-garbage-out (GIGO) exercise. Jerome Kassirer, a former editor of *NEJM*, summarizes the ways corporations bake positive results into their studies in *On the Take* (2004).

> *Some… intentionally compare their new drugs to placebo controls when the appropriate control is the best available treatment. Comparisons can also be staged between the new drug and a drug that is not a perfect fit with the symptoms in question. Doses of comparison drugs can be rigged to favor a new drug, and duration of treatment can be carefully selected to favor a new drug… Frequently… the investigator['s]… proposal must be approved first by the company's marketing division… Industry sponsored research [may then] withhold information… [or] keep results secret.*

The first principle of research is, *Does this make sense?* Much of medical knowledge does not need statistical study. Fixing a dislocated shoulder is an example. It is a cure, and the pain vanishes. The short-term benefit of morphine, used for centuries, is also obvious. At one time, penicillin for pneumonia worked for nearly every patient.

Physicians believe in randomized controlled trials at the expense of common sense, according to Gordon Smith, who composed a parody about it. He says that we have not yet performed randomized controlled studies for parachutes. Such a test would involve a control group without parachutes. He suggested in his 2003 *BMJ* editorial, "Parachute use to prevent death and major trauma related to gravitational challenge: systematic review of randomised controlled trials," that the most rabid advocates of statistical science should be the control group for this trial.

Charlie Poole, a professor of statistics and epidemiology at the University of North Carolina, agrees. He said, "Controlled trials, which began as a means of protecting patients from the biases of doctors, have become instead a method to enhance business in great part because drug companies have managed to hook doctors to the crack pipe of statistical significance." David Healy adds, "statistical significance should be abandoned immediately and universally."

These observers understand the math. They can tell the proper calculations from the bad ones by reading an article. They cannot be sure what went into the calculations, however. This may include manipulation and concealment. It is the "garbage in." Academics know all too well that they may fool readers in GIGO situations. Common sense, total disclosure, and eliminating industry funding are necessary to make the medical literature valuable again.

3) "Data torturing" or "data mining" is statistical trickery that ruins conclusions. Here is how this works. After a study is complete, computer analysis is used to examine "relationships." Gigantic studies have many variables, such as patient age, sex, different diagnoses, and so forth. This makes mathematical correlations by chance alone inevitable.

Statistical significance is supposedly credible if there is

only one chance in twenty of a relationship happening fortuitously. But if a thousand relationships are studied, as would be the case with 32 variables, 50, which is one in twenty, will appear to have a significant connection by chance alone. These meaningless random links would be different if the study was repeated.

The author who performs data torture then describes these 50 fake relationships as real. Phony retrospective studies like this are common. They are meaningless exercises whose purpose is to promote products and careers.

Watershed material is rare. But researchers must publish breakthroughs so they can attract attention and get more money. Editors always need to print something interesting with new conclusions. These conspirators call this "subset analysis," a pseudoscientific name used to disguise the fraud.

Honest researchers define what is being looked for *before* the investigation begins and stick with it. Treatments that are true successes are rare but visible. They do not need armies of study subjects sweated over by Ph.D. mathematicians. Unfortunately for academics, most studies are negative—the therapies do not work.

4) The FDA now permits "surrogate" or "soft" endpoints for drug approval studies. These include blood sugar, blood pressure, bone density, cholesterol, tumor size reduction, and disease-free survival. Their advantage is that numbers like these are easy to tabulate and study.

"Hard" endpoints include death, blindness, stroke, or bone fracture. No equivocation is possible for death. For example, in cancer treatment, if fatality rates are unchanged, measuring chemotherapy response using tumor size reduction is useless. Stroke, heart attack rates, or even total hospital days seem like reasonable benchmarks, but if the death rate is unchanged, the patient benefits are doubtful.

In psychiatry, nearly all measures are surrogate except things such as suicide rate or premature deaths because of the

—considerable—drug toxicity. Their studies are based almost entirely on questionnaires and observations, both of which are subjective measures.

We treat diabetes to help people live longer. In people with type II, pills are sometimes used to control blood sugar, which is a surrogate outcome. Reducing this number has never been proven to decrease stroke or heart attack, the major causes of death for diabetics. Theirs is a complicated problem with many unknown factors, not a simple issue of blood sugar control.

A 2008 *NEJM* trial, "Effects of Intensive Glucose Lowering in Type 2 Diabetes" studied oral sugar drugs. The investigators found that there were *more* deaths in the group that used higher doses and had lower blood sugars. These medications sometimes cause fatal hypoglycemia and other adverse effects. Aggressive sugar lowering may not be beneficial, especially for those over 50. One of the three new classes of oral glucose drugs does not decrease death rates at all.

Even corporate employees from companies that are contracted to study drugs point out problems with surrogate endpoints. Scientists from Nuventra wrote in their blog that arbitrarily chosen numbers sometimes do not relate to patient outcomes. They remind us that rigorous post-marketing studies are needed if we permit surrogate outcomes. Unfortunately, after-market trials are not an FDA priority. Instead, they wait for the patient harms to occur. This is mostly after the profits have been made.

Using "combined" or "composite" endpoints: In trials of cardiac stents, the calculations may lump together both deaths and the need for future stents. This is a logical fallacy. Why should a stent be placed to avoid another stent? Combined endpoints are mathematical deceptions unless the variables are analyzed independently.

Endpoint selection is also critical. If these are improper, studies may legitimize toxic, ineffective, and horrifically expensive medications and therapies. One sign of a worthless endpoint is that the patient doesn't notice any improvement until told about it by the doctor[1].

CONCLUSIONS

COVID-19 explained using doctor math: In mid-2020, my friend Stan Cohen is terrified of Coronavirus, and he plies us with horrifying stories. Although he is a professional with a graduate degree, statistics are not his specialty. Stan and everyone else are being tutored by talking heads who know no more math than a house cat.

The pundits throw around *surrogate* disease measures such as testing results, hospitalizations, and infection rates. These measures distort conclusions for several reasons. First, the COVID test identifies only half of those with active disease. Second, people briefly infected with a minor or asymptomatic variant seldom get tested. Third, the numbers of tests being done has increased, so we are identifying more and more of these inconsequential cases along with some who have already recovered. There is no way to be sure any of these surrogates are valid without purposefully infecting and then studying a sizable group, which is too dangerous.

The only reliable, hard endpoint to evaluate the pandemic is *deaths due to the disease*. Although this may be confounded by factors either way, it is what we care about most. It is not a questionable surrogate—we can count bodies. But even this figure may be distorted, propped up by political machinations. It is hard to be sure.

Deaths due to other seasonal viral illnesses give us some perspective. These kill 291,000 to 646,000 people worldwide every year. Also, pandemics occur every few decades:

COVID (by Oct 2020):881,000 deaths
Flu pandemic 2009:284,000 deaths (CDC)
Hong Kong flu (1968):1-4 million deaths
Asian flu (1956-8):1.5-2 million deaths
Spanish flu (1918-9):20-50 m deaths

Even death numbers, however, are just the *relative risk of dying from COVID alone*. Every day, 8,000 pass away in the US and 156,000 die worldwide. Violence, suicide, and many other complex factors are in play; the current pandemic is only one variable and not the biggest one. Restricted access to medical care might *decrease* mortality.

This fatality rate from all causes, the all-important *absolute* fatalities, is likely unaffected by Coronavirus, lost in statistical "noise" or variation. Since COVID primarily affects the elderly and the infirm, many people are just dying a few months early. No one denies that this is an aggressive disease, but the total fatalities from all causes might be the same or close to the same in 2020 as any other year.

The media brainwashes us with surrogates instead of the hard endpoint of death, and they spout relative risk rather than absolute risk—the identical deceptions used by medical journals. It is all done for the money. The press uses panic to sell advertising and the journals use lies to sell drugs.

We cannot blame bad research entirely on corporations. John Ioannidis wrote about "publication bias," the tendency for journals to print news of recent findings and ignore or not publish boring stories of negative studies lacking exciting outcomes. He wrote, "For most study designs and settings, it is more likely for a research claim to be false than true." This is not conflict of interest or supported medical industries trying to develop false evidence for profitable drugs and devices. He is saying the publication process itself is flawed.

The most troubling part of this story is that journal editors do not speak up. They know they are using deceptive math to approve products that do not work. Canadian academic nephrologist and commentator, Jason Fung, summarizes:

> *Does the CEO of Philip Morris (maker of Marlboro cigarettes) smoke? That tells you all you need to know about the health risks.*

> *Do the editors of the NEJM and the Lancet believe [evidence-based medicine] anymore? Not at all. So neither should we. We can't believe evidence-based medicine until the evidence has been cleaned up from the corrupting influence of commercial interests.*

A committee of readers should sanction journal editors every time they disgrace themselves by publishing data torturing (subset analysis). We should question surrogate endpoint studies, and we must abandon NNTs over 50. Allowing discussion of relative risk without including the absolute risk in a paper's abstract should get a journal editor fired. These publications cause hundreds of billions of wasted dollars and hundreds of thousands of deaths. The editors know what they are doing; they do it for the money, and they fool nearly everyone.

CHAPTER 23

PATIENT TIPS TO LEARN THE TRUTH

If you don't know where you are going, all roads will get you there.

— NORTIN HADLER, MD

―――――

WHERE SHOULD YOU GET INFORMATION, and whom can you trust? I learned that the reason ordinary blog authors produce unreferenced junk is that they must compose ten a day. They don't care whether they are right or wrong because their success is measured by the number of eyeballs passing over their drivel rather than accuracy. Correcting mistakes later gets them even more traffic.

The lay press typically concocts an "experts disagree" story, which is the proper way to write about nebulous social and political issues. It is the wrong way to analyze science, even the pretend science of healthcare.

Medical blogs and journals are worse in some ways than click-bait blogs. I studied the NEJM and others for decades as if they were biblical, but learned only recently about the ghostwriting, faked studies, and sales pitches. The barrier to understanding this was that they seemed so credible and authoritative.

Can you trust anyone? "Meta-analysis" journal articles are the best we have. They amalgamate major studies and try to come to conclusions. Cochrane does the finest job despite their recent lapses with the HPV vaccine and clot-dissolving drugs.

The Mayo Clinic website might be the top resource for patients. Wikipedia also has an excellent reputation. See the *References and Resources* at the end of this book as well. If you dive into medical journals, the *BMJ* might be the most reliable. And a paper's abstract may tell you enough to decide whether to spend your time looking at the rest.

Knowledge is power. You or your advocates can use google as well as any doctor. Diagnoses may be hidden to your providers because they are busy. Doctors have an expression: "If it quacks, it is likely a duck." This simple rule says that the common things are more probable than rare ones (this is "Occam's Razor"). But also keep in mind that if you are forced to research, your doctors might have missed something unusual.

I still cannot resist the occasional Google search for medical information, and I confess to sometimes reading the abstracts in the first three links. When I quoted a study to one of my peers recently, she chided me that it was likely put together by some pharmaceutical company. I resented being called out, but when I checked the disclosures at the end of the article, I found that the manufacturer had funded it.

Recap: never forget the three clues:

✪ If you cannot understand something, it is likely a lie or a sales pitch.

✪ Always check the end of the article for the funding disclosures.

✪ If there are huge numbers, or there is an NNT over 100, or "we need further studies," or there are editorials about conflicting data, your conclusion is easy. The therapy is worthless.

PART V

PHYSICIANS ON THE TAKE

CHAPTER 24

REAL DOCTORS ARE WITH US
STILL

ATTORNEYS, business people, and others frequently have high skills and work hard, but top doctors are in a class of their own. In a bygone era, Alexander Fleming refused to patent penicillin, and Jonas Salk did the same with the polio vaccine. The spirit of these and other forebears survives in our finest physicians. Here are a few stories about them.

Pediatricians' pay is the lowest of any specialty. They view their responsibility so seriously that they refuse to take advantage of their beloved patients. Money is a distant consideration for them.

Oncologists perform occasional miracles. They may improve or cure sick patients who have rare diseases by using careful combinations of medications. A beautiful woman I call Baby Bear was 20 when she rapidly developed lumps on her forehead and upper eyelid. The doctors biopsied them. It was a rare, aggressive malignant sarcoma that responds poorly to chemotherapy. If this is discovered on a leg or arm, an amputation is often performed. Baby's doctors considered extensive surgery, including removal of her eye.

On our advice, Baby's mom sent the microscopic findings

to top US pathologists who referred her to an oncologist who came out of retirement to help her. He had seen six other cases like this, and four of them had responded to a unique chemotherapy drug combination he invented. With this, her tumors gradually shrank. She had an eyelid surgery that went well, and she kept her eye. Three years later, she is tumor free and still beautiful.

I learned as a trainee that cardiologists and cardiac surgeons do jobs that were too tough for me. They save lives, counsel the dying, and must always be gentle and sympathetic when dealing with families, which might be the hardest part. They shoulder responsibilities that keep them awake and functioning for days on end with only a few hours sleep. Only a high-energy, insomniac polymath can do this right. Much of the science supporting their work has dissolved, but these people are still exceptional individuals who have many skills.

General surgeons save lives using procedures routine for them, such as appendectomy. When they operate, they have to be emotionally indifferent to the possibility of an error; if they worried about it, they could never pick up a scalpel. This strength is sometimes at odds with the interpersonal skills required by the rest of their environment.

With the slightest misstep, nursing staff and administrators may criticize specialists like these. I know a brilliant general surgeon who trained in the military and left as a colonel. He works day and night, 85 hours a week. Some of his surgeries pay only $400, and this includes all the hours of postoperative care. His wife cleans his office because she feels they can barely afford a housekeeper. Since he has a hard time suffering fools, his hospital nursing staff forced him to spend 20 of his precious hours on "sensitivity training."

Many doctors think orthopedists are stupid. True, they are not experts in standard internal medicine. But the best of them are familiar with a seemingly endless array of bone, joint, and soft tissue problems, and display judgment and restraint about when to operate and when to hold off. Top orthopedists have intellect, integrity, and manual skills. They also work long hours.

Neurosurgeons are not just the best surgeons in the hospital—they are usually the best physicians. They must be the master of multiple fields: neurology, some oncology, critical care medicine, and much internal medicine. If they deviate a few millimeters during many of their operations, the patient might die or have brain damage. Their surgeries sometimes last 20 hours. (My rule was that two hours were enough for me.) They need the nerves of a combat general, for they must take agonizing risks.

Brain aneurysms are an example. These are arteries with localized weaknesses and ballooning which may rupture spontaneously and cause a stroke or death. Delicate operations, which are fatal in 2.5% of cases, are used to prevent this. In another 10%, the patient is left with permanent disability. The surgeon must be emotionally detached or they cannot do the work. Worse, neurosurgeons are routinely called to evaluate people whose aneurysm has already ruptured and bled into their brain. Here, the chances of permanent disability or death may be more likely than recovery, even if they perform the operation.

The pressure of poor results is constant. Neurosurgeons must counsel some patients that they inevitably will do poorly, and others must be told they are dying. Neurosurgeons require megalomania and a touch of genius. They may have strained interactions with staff. If you need one, pay attention, try to keep your mouth shut, and if there is an issue with the bedside manner, ignore it. You are meeting someone with special abilities.

I could tell many other stories of exceptional physicians,

but they are not my subject. As you go through their industry in the following chapters, try to bring to mind the device and drug company settlements with their gross revenue figures. Remember the insurance companies as well. I will soon introduce you to hospitals. Physician theft is amateurish compared with these bandits.

CHAPTER 25

SCIENCE DEBUNKED THE HEART DOCTORS

How much can a patient be expected to do, anyway? Caveat emptor may be an appropriate slogan for selling used cars or life insurance, but it is not a worthy dictum for health care. In the final analysis, it is not a patient's responsibility to protect himself against the medical profession; it is the profession's responsibility to protect the patient.

— JEROME KASSIRER, MD, *ON THE TAKE (2005)*

CORONARY ARTERY DISEASE (CAD) is blockage of the arteries supplying the heart with blood. It is the top cause of death in the US. When it happens suddenly, people get heart attacks, which damage the heart muscle, and they may die. We have high-tech weapons to treat this problem, but over the past few decades, studies have proven that they are nearly complete failures.

Coronary artery bypass grafting (CABG) heart surgery is sewing new blood vessels on the heart to permit blood to flow around blocked areas. This logically appealing, plumbing-type solution was first performed in the 1960s. The second approach, angioplasty, is a more recent development.

Wires and tiny balloons are used to pry the arteries open. Mesh tubes called stents hold them open. This is often done while a heart attack is occurring.

The first step in the modern approach is to identify people who have the disease and might get a heart attack. We ask patients about chest pain and "cardiac risk factors." These include smoking, diabetes, cholesterol, high blood pressure, and family history. Being overweight and male are also risks.

If doctors are suspicious that the coronary arteries are partially blocked, they often have the patient do a "stress test." This is a walk on a treadmill while the doctor checks the heart's function using an EKG. Sometimes, imaging is used to look at the anatomy during this exercise. If heart disease seems likely, the patient then gets referred for "angiography" to see if there is a blockage. For this, the cardiologist squirts dye directly into the coronary arteries and takes x-rays.

Patients with chest pain have stress-testing if their story and examination suggest heart problems. Those with suspicious stress tests and the ones who seem sick get an angiogram. After this, the doctors may consider surgery or angioplasty, depending on the situation. If the first treatment fails, the doctor will usually pass the patient to the other specialist for the alternative treatment.

We perform stress testing nearly universally, but its predictive power is little better than a coin toss. Doing them does not improve survival. Radiologic imaging during stress testing is of little benefit, either. These tests are wrong twice as often as they are right. They often detect a 50 percent blockage, which is a routine finding that is a poor predictor of future death. This needs no invasive treatment.

CABG surgery is proven to lengthen life *only* for the tiny fraction of patients who have severe left main coronary artery blockage. This is a one-centimeter vessel which feeds two of the three primary heart arteries. It divides into a Y, supplying their inflow, then the blood goes through these into most of the rest of the heart. Significant obstruction in this tiny spot is found in only three (3) percent of all heart attacks.

After a CABG plumbing-job around this small section, eighty-five percent of patients will be alive five years later, but only 65 percent of them will survive five years if they just take medications. *This twenty (20) percent improvement in survival at five years for this small group is the entire benefit—for all CABAG surgeries.* Sewing artery bypasses around other areas of artery obstructions does *not* improve lifespan.

The whole multibillion-dollar skyscraper of coronary artery bypass surgery was built on this slender foundation. No studies have ever shown other justifications. As early as 1989, a Veterans Administration trial found that cardiac bypass surgery did not improve overall five-year survival more than merely taking medications. Fewer people died of heart disease when they get the operations, but they did not live longer on average because they died of other things— including presumably the operation itself.

There are enormous, teetering wings of the heart surgery machine with no foundation at all. These include the claim that doing a complicated surgery to bypass blockages in all three coronaries works as effectively as bypassing the left main artery alone. Although operating on this "left main equivalent" situation seems reasonable, the studies have proven that triple vessel surgery does not extend life.

The gorillas in the CABG room are the complications. Two to nine percent of the people getting the surgery die immediately, and about a third—some studies say half—of those surviving have significant, measurable brain damage. Angioplasty, in contrast, has few such issues, and the fatalities are only a fraction of a percent when performed for patients who are not having a heart attack. The cardiologists tout it as the safe way to treat CAD[1].

The studies which debunked angioplasty and stents were as unforeseen and staggering as the ones deflating

CABG surgery. In 2007, the NEJM published the "COURAGE" trial of over 2000 patients (study authors like acronyms; this one somehow stands for "Clinical Outcomes Utilizing Revascularization and Aggressive Drug Evaluation"). It showed that neither stents nor angioplasty improved survival or subsequent heart attack rates in patients with stable coronary artery disease.

A follow-up report by these COURAGE authors showed improvements in angina and a few qualities of life measures, but these effects lasted less than 36 months. Based on this slender support, the operations continued. The cardiologists thought it was reasonable because stent deaths are so rare.

Finally, the ORBITA study showed conclusively that these procedures were without survival benefit for stable cardiac disease—in people who were not having a heart attack. Neither pain nor chances of further heart attacks decreased either. This trial used an invasive "sham" or faked procedure for the control group, which is the most definitive type of surgical evaluation. There were only 230 patients, but the results were indisputable[2].

Drug "eluting" stents leak drugs into the surrounding area, but they did not help patient survival either and cause an increase in blood clots. The science was clear: stents and angioplasty in routine care do not improve outcomes.

In 2019, a federally funded trial again discredited over 90 percent, possibly over 95 percent, of the cardiology and cardiac surgical invasive procedures. The researchers treated 5000 patients with stable heart disease with either CABG or stents. Neither therapy improved lifespan or heart attacks when compared to diet and drugs. These patients were not those who were having heart attacks at the time of the interventions. The researchers also excluded those with left main coronary artery disease.

Just as for CABG surgery, there is one narrow case where stents supposedly work. This is during a severe heart attack when the EKG has a pattern called "ST-elevation myocardial infarction" or STEMI. This is a complete or near-complete coronary artery blockage. When stents are placed during STEMIs, the cardiologists proclaim they save one person in 40, a number needed to treat of 40.

The American Heart Association and many others world-wide market this as "intervening during the golden hour" (lately they have been promoting this more for strokes). Patients in their most vulnerable state, often in severe pain, get rushed from the emergency department to the catheterization lab and treated with angioplasty and stents. They are incapable of making reasoned decisions. Nortin Hadler summarizes: "Stenting belongs to one of the bleakest chapters in the history of Western medicine… Cardiologists are marching on because the interventional cardiology industry has a cash flow comparable to the GDP of many countries."

The latest marketing ploy is to remind the public about "atypical" pain, which is serious but unlike the usual, distinctive heart attack pain patterns. People are now racing to the hospital, into this dysfunctional system, if they have any twinge in their chest.

Angioplasty causes strokes, heart attacks, rhythm disturbances, and bleeding. Are more STEMI heart attack patients saved by angioplasty during a heart attack than are killed by the procedure? When performed during a heart attack:

ANGIOPLASTY SAVES: 1/40, or 2.5%
ANGIOPLASTY FATALITIES: 1/167 to 1/43: .6% to 2.3%
ANGIOPLASTY COMPLICATIONS: 1/50, or 2%

Does the 1/40 "saved" figure already take into account the people who die from the procedure? I do not think it makes any difference, given the entire picture, but if you still have doubts, ask your cardiologist. I doubt if they could convince me.

If we could forget the cardiologists' conflict of interest and believe that their numbers made sense, the expense of doing angioplasties on 40 people to save one is 40 x the $35,000 cost, $1.4 million. Since heart attack patients have an average age in their late 60s, the number of years of life being bought is uncertain. There are many other ways to spend this money that would do more good and save more years of life.

In the US, at least 85 percent (the lowest figure I could find) of coronary angioplasties are performed on patients who have uncomplicated, stable chest pain, *where there is no chance of success.*

To justify the process, cardiologists often send their patients through the emergency room, saying that they have "unstable angina." This means chest pain occurring without physical exertion, not relieved by resting or medication, which may be worsening. Since it is a judgment call with an imprecise definition, this diagnosis gets abused. I spoke to emergency physicians in 2019, who confirmed that they saw this scenario frequently.

Note: when angioplasty is done like this as an "elective procedure," for no patient benefit, and not during a heart attack, it thankfully only kills .2 percent or 1/500.

———

CONCLUSIONS

How can treating cardiologists and surgeons condone all this? Surgeons rarely look at statistical evidence. They say they see the heart coming alive when the blood comes back after they sew on new arteries. They support CABG surgeries based on their specialty's authority.

Cardiologists continue to place stents long after the studies proved they were ineffective. They say they have cases every week where there is an immediate decrease in chest pain after stent placement. My attempts to interview several of them about the statistics were met with hostility.

The University of California San Francisco cardiologist

Rita Redberg said, "It's just like a sugar pill. We know sugar pills make a lot of people feel better — though sugar procedures make even more people feel even better." Dr. Katz agrees: *Placebos work avidly for pain, especially placebo surgery.*

Doctors are only human. Upton Sinclair explains: "It is difficult to get a man to understand something when his salary depends on his not understanding it." Doctors do care for their patients, but because they are getting paid, they have trouble reconciling issues like this.

How many of these procedures get done? Although CABG surgery has been declining somewhat for nearly 20 years, about a half-million still get performed annually in the US. At about the same time, each year, a million angioplasties are done, and about a million patients had stents placed (2013, 2018).

In the US, angioplasty and stents cost $20,000 to $50,000, while CABG surgery is $70,000 to $200,000. CABG is about $28,000 in the UK if not covered by insurance. The US yearly bill for all stents is roughly $12 billion, and for CABG surgeries, the total is about the same. US cardiovascular disease, including stroke, costs nearly a billion dollars a day, including lost productivity (CDC).

Proper diet and exercise must be vital for healthy hearts, but just what is optimal is unknown. Exercise helps, but the studies are unclear. Michael Greger has a comprehensive website summarizing thousands of studies that support vegan or non-animal diets. He presents plausible evidence that these diets improve and sometimes even cure heart disease. He is also concerned about animal rights, which may bias his opinions.

Bill Clinton had coronary artery bypass and stents for severe heart disease. His problem went away after he began a vegetable diet. This sounds convincing but is only an anecdote.

Despite many studies, there is no consensus whether

vegans live longer. These diets do seem to improve disease specific or *relative* risk of coronary artery disease but do not improve the *absolute* or all-causes chance of dying.

Jason Fung credibly touts higher fat diets and fasting. He says that when people fast, their metabolism or internal caloric consumption stays high, which aids weight loss. By comparison, ordinary calorie-restricted diets *lower* metabolic levels, which is a big disadvantage. After this sort of dieting, it may be a permanent or near-permanent effect. Fung says his patients lower their cholesterol, eliminate diabetes, and discontinue most drugs.

Scientific proof is imperfect for any diet. John Ioannidis, the renowned Stanford study design expert, says that most trials of diet and health are flawed. They are too small, not randomized, or otherwise biased. Both of the two diets above restrict calories; this may be responsible for the benefits.

The US has showered money and prestige on our heart doctors, who in return oversee our second most expensive and ineffective medical specialty after mental health. Our national obsession with these high technologies has distracted us from the possibility of more straightforward solutions. Other first-world countries perform heart procedures at a fraction of our rate. They get less doctoring, which could be the reason their citizens live longer.

CHAPTER 26

SURGERY: MONEY BEFORE PATIENTS

Most of the high-ticket items (procedures and pharmaceuticals) are
minimally effective or ineffective. Many of these are considered
standards of care. Many are cash cows, touted by vested interests.

— Nortin Hadler, MD, Worried Sick (2010)

The hard evidence for surgical care ranges from speculative to nonexistent. The field is almost unstudied; we rely on tradition; we give surgeons near-complete therapeutic autonomy, and many of their net outcomes are in doubt. A few quality trials, such as arthroscopic knee sham-surgery studies, are finally emerging.

The fee-for-service system pays physicians for each service and doing surgery pays the most. This conflict of interest often causes patient harm.

Our back pain therapies cost over $100 billion a year, yet they do not work. This is more than the spending on all the US police forces of the towns, cities, counties, and states added together. These treatments include hot packs, ultrasound, chiropractors, acupuncture, laser therapy, steroid injections, spinal surgeries, opioid painkillers, electrical stimulation, and osteopathic manipulation. None of these improves pain over the long term.

Cathryn Jakobson Ramin, motivated by her own pain, came to this conclusion after spending six years investigating the industry[1]. Nortin Hadler, MD, had the same opinion: "For back pain, there are over 300 randomized controlled trials testing pharmaceuticals, advice as to activity, various gadgets, and many physical [therapy] modalities without a hint of a benefit[2]."

These treatments create chronic dependency on expensive procedures and providers. The physical therapists call their traditional treatments "shake and bake." This refers to hooking patients up to heaters, vibrators, or electric stimulators, and then aggressively billing insurance. The business model is like the chiropractors, who have no more support for their treatments than the rest of the industry. Yet they are trained to recommend frequent, virtually indefinite follow-up, calling it "internal marketing."

Expensive imaging studies are used to justify surgery, but despite this, the reasons for back pain are rarely clear. Nearly everyone over 50, healthy or not, has radiologic abnormalities, but few scan findings have a definite relationship to the cause(s) of back pain.

However, surgeons get paid for operating, chiropractors get paid for manipulation and doing x-rays, and physical therapists get paid for their noninvasive methods. They are all able to convince themselves they are doing excellent work.

Tylenol, aspirin, and ibuprofen-type drugs ease pain. But according to Ramin's review, specialized, directed exercise is the only treatment that works for back pain. An adequately trained physical therapist can supervise it. Patients must sometimes work out for months through the pain to produce improvement. After years of frustration with wretched surgical outcomes, a few surgeons have abandoned their lucrative practices and opened rehabilitation clinics.

Some studies show no difference between physical therapy and surgery, and spinal fusion surgery does not improve pain consistently enough to be worth the risk. It is an unscrupulous $12 billion a year industry in the US. Each procedure may cost up to $100,000. The workers compensation industry supports it by reimbursing more than other insurers. Litigation is part of the game, and this finances yet another "stakeholder" group feeding off our healthcare dollars, the lawyers.

Back pain is the leading cause of disability worldwide. Surgery is an enormous part of it, and it is often accompanied by opioid dependence. Only fifteen percent of patients getting spinal fusion surgery for pain ever return to work. The direct costs are the ninth highest of all US medical conditions. Nortin Hadler says, "So many high-ticket items that are trumpeted as the triumphs of US medicine are little more than a scam. Spine surgery for regional low back pain has earned this ignominy."

A huge Cochrane review questioned the use of surgery for spinal stenosis, even though the experts accept this as a reasonable indication to operate. Cochrane said there was a "paucity of evidence on the efficacy of surgery for lumbar spinal stenosis, as to date, no trials have compared surgery with no treatment, placebo or sham surgery." Translated: we have no reason to believe it works.

Spinal fusion procedures are much overused, but there are a few compelling reasons to try them despite the poor quality of the studies. Nerve entrapment may produce weakness in an arm or leg, or create bowel or bladder problems. Patients who have a fever (infection), weight loss (cancer), or other worrisome signs must be evaluated carefully. But pain and radiologic findings alone are typically used to justify surgery. This is without foundation.

The money is so colossal and passed out so freely that it has attracted criminals. The biggest fraud in California history involved back surgeries. Michael Drobot, a hospital owner, colluded with orthopedic surgeons to kick back money for people referring these procedures to his group. They paid $10,000 for each referral, and they eventually gave out $40 million in total inducements. They even bribed state legislators.

The surgeons billed each operation for about $250,000, and by the end, insurance companies paid $600 million. Drobot, who was 72 in 2018, went to prison for five years.

The good news is that back surgery is somewhat falling out of favor. As recently as 2010, orthopedic conventions were still lavish parties hosted by Medtronic and other hardware manufacturers. Recently, Medtronic has cut the funding, and the meetings are duller.

A neurosurgeon's counterpoint follows. He says that in a few special cases, back surgery helps.

> Using the right surgeon matters... a lot. The best of us only consider operating on patients whose pain radiates down a leg or arm and is accompanied by numbness and/or weakness. We try to wait four to six months to see if the syndrome cures itself, but if things are getting worse, we occasionally operate sooner. We only work on the spinal segment that hurts. This process, carefully implemented, has the best chance of excellent results. Greedy back surgeons operate even when there is no numbness, weakness, or radiation accompanying the pain. They do not wait several months to see if the problem goes away before doing surgery, and many do additional procedures on nearby spine areas that have scan abnormalities but do not hurt. For their patients, the procedure isn't the solution for back pain—it is the start of a lifetime of disability.

Endoscopic knee surgery performed for arthritis pain and torn cartilage is useless. Sham operation studies have debunked it. Investigators compared patients who had the surgery with patients who only had incisions and anesthesia. On average, the two groups had the same pain relief. Some observers believe that the patients who get operated on have worse outcomes because the surgeons remove cartilage padding. The orthopedists have been quibbling about these results, but they are still performing thousands of cases. It is a $4 billion a year industry in the US.

Here is how it works. Your knee hurts. You go to an orthopedist. You have an MRI scan costing between $800 and $3000, or possibly more if the surgeon owns the machine. The radiologist sees the natural age-related fragmentation of cartilage pads between the big knee bones and describes it in their report.

The orthopedist recommends a $5000 arthroscopic procedure to "clean it up." Surgicenter charges can be $40,000 or more if the surgeon has an aggressive biller. Your insurance company lets them get away with it.

You spend a half-hour in the operating room, and your knee is sore for a few weeks. It usually gets better. Some get worse and require more painkillers later because of the cartilage removal. Patients and surgeons both fool themselves because a placebo, especially a surgical placebo, works well for pain.

Your orthopedist refers you to a physical therapist who might work for them. The bill is thousands of dollars if you have good insurance.

Note: there are reasons to do endoscopic knee surgery, such as a knee that locks. Orthopedics is an art, just like the rest of medicine. HMOs do not profit by doing more operations, so many of them do not offer this procedure unless a patient pressures the doctor.

Most total hip replacements are successful. Many people who could not walk are pain free or nearly pain-free after surgery. Most patients go home the same day. Even though there has never been a proper study, it works.

Think twice before agreeing to total knee replacement, however. Up to 40 percent of patients require at least as many painkillers after the operation. Some start on new medicines during the year following the surgery. Other studies describe pain persisting for three to five years. Twenty percent have chronic pain.

Fifteen percent of knee replacements fail before five years and need another procedure. Orthopedists usually state the results the other way: 85 percent last over a decade, and most patients have pain relief. They remind me that complete rehabilitation may take a year or two. An excellent *Kaiser Health News* article summarizes these issues with references and adds that some believe the procedure is overused. Despite these doubts, I know a half-dozen people who had a total knee replacement, and every one of them is pain-free and functional. If you have so much pain that you consider a total knee surgery, find a surgeon with experience.

Outsiders have questioned the surgical numbers of obstetrics and gynecology for decades. This specialty may have saved more lives since 1950 than any other because of improved care during childbirth. Despite this remarkable contribution, I have heard about their high surgical numbers since the 1980s.

One in three US women has their uterus removed before they are 60, the highest rate in the industrialized world. Our surgeons perform six hundred thousand hysterectomies each year, and both ovaries also get removed in 44 percent. Some gynecologists tell women they do not need their uteri and ovaries except to conceive. Nobody tells a man of any age he doesn't need his testicles.

The usual excuse for doing a total hysterectomy, which includes the ovaries, is to prevent ovarian cancer. This is reasoning by people with no grasp of doctor-math. The procedure cuts out only the one percent lifelong chance of dying from ovarian cancer. The relative risk for ovarian cancer becomes zero.

Unfortunately, there are many more deaths overall after ovary removal. Not only does one patient die from the procedure every 500 cases, but worse—the missing hormones no longer protect women from breast cancer, heart disease, osteoporosis, and other issues.

In the natural change of life, with the ovarian decline, hormone production decreases but does not go away completely. If their ovaries are removed, however, women crash into a dramatic, unpleasant, complete menopause. This is castration: the hormones sustaining the mood and many physical functions are missing.

Hysterectomy procedures are fast and pay reasonably well. Gynecologists sometimes perform hysterectomies for bleeding that is inconvenient but not serious. An open hysterectomy through the belly may take just a half-hour. Recoveries are easier if the surgeon uses an endoscope, but this is a longer operation.

Sometimes it is worth it. For example, benign fibroid uterine overgrowth occurs in about 75 percent of women during their lives, and they occasionally bleed. When there is severe bleeding and pain, the procedure often gets an excellent result. After a hysterectomy, some patients find that their sexual relations improve.

However, hysterectomy is a shock that can damage or destroy ovarian function even when they are left behind. Studies by Masters and Johnson relate an intact uterus and cervix to orgasm, and some studies show fewer after their removal. There are many patient stories about sexual decline after the procedure, even when the ovaries are left.

My patients have told me about this. The procedure threw some of them into menopause in their mid-30s after a hysterectomy without ovary removal. I checked their

234 I BUTCHERED BY "HEALTHCARE"

hormone blood tests, and they were low, which explained the hot flashes and other symptoms.

Conservative treatments may cure many non-cancerous conditions. These include endometrial ablation, which is the surgical destruction of the interior of the womb through the cervix. This stops certain types of bleeding. Gynecologists can also remove excess uterine tissue with an endoscope. However, uterine fibroid removal without hysterectomy often requires lengthy, complicated operations. Most gynecologists hate these procedures. Uterine artery embolization is blockage of the uterine artery with injected material. This is an attempt to shrink the uterus by cutting off part of its blood supply. Proper counseling about these options is uncommon.

Stanley West, a prominent New York gynecologist, says that 90 percent of hysterectomies are unnecessary (2002). Other experts (2008) say that two out of three hysterectomies are unwarranted. Surgeons do not always offer alternatives. Only ten percent of hysterectomies are performed for previously diagnosed cancers of the uterus, ovaries, or fallopian tubes. Pathologists say a full third of the wombs and ovaries they examine after surgery are entirely normal. There was no reason they could find for the operation.

Since surgical indications are not standardized, different parts of the country have different hysterectomy rates. Regional variation in surgical numbers is evidence of overuse. Hysterectomy Educational Resources and Services (HERS) is a group that aims to make sure every woman considering a uterus operation thoroughly understands it. They say the gynecologists vastly overuse hysterectomy, and that the counseling is nearly always inadequate.

This group keeps a registry of ailments following hysterectomies. These include incontinence, sexual dysfunction, premature menopause, and pelvic problems of various kinds. Women who go to gynecologists recommended by HERS avoid surgery two-thirds of the time.

Written consent forms are the general standard for elective surgery in the US, but some gynecologic organizations oppose them. They claim that every situation is different. Several states, including California, passed laws that mandated written consent for hysterectomy. Physicians believe that legislating medical practice is not desirable, but this seems reasonable in this case in view of the circumstances.

The surgeons perform too many cesarean sections as well. Each year in the US, they perform 1.3 million, a third of births. It is the most common major surgery in America. Only cataract implants, which are medically trivial, are done more often. The World Health Organization says cesareans should be performed in only ten to fifteen percent of deliveries. Doing more saves no lives.

Maternal death rates after a cesarean are about six times those after vaginal delivery, although both are low. The operation costs, including hospital expenses, are five to ten times more than an ordinary birth. There are other disadvantages. Surgical recoveries are much longer and more painful than vaginal births. Sometimes the pain lasts weeks. Blood clots and infections are more likely, and surgical anesthesia is yet another risk. Even the obstetricians concede that over half of these operations are unneeded. But pregnant women are a kind of science-free zone because randomized controlled trials are tough to get approved. It is hard to be sure what is optimal.

Episiotomy is cutting the back of a woman's vagina to facilitate delivery. Studies show it neither decreases pain nor cesarean section rate. This procedure has become less common, but there are geographical areas where gynecologists perform it at five times the national average. Insurance pays for it.

Laparoscopic gallbladder removal was invented in 1985 and came into heavy usage in the early 1990s. Surgeons use lighted scopes and small instruments inserted through holes in the abdomen instead of cutting a long incision. Since post-operative pain is much less, the procedure usually requires only one night's hospitalization. With the open method, a week is usual.

After this invention, gallbladder procedures in the US immediately increased by almost half, as expected in a "free market" with insurance reimbursement. About 300,000 get done every year. But while 20 million people in the US have gallstones, the majority never get symptoms. Surgeons frequently perform the operation for minimal or no obvious indication, with the idea that problems are being prevented. They are given wide latitude. Neither the FDA nor any other regulatory body formally oversees them.

Since they use the surgery for nearly any symptom, it is now hard to find patients treated medically for comparison. Fortunately, at Johns Hopkins, a study of 17,000 people with biliary pancreatitis gave us some insights. Seventy-eight percent of them had their gallbladders removed within 30 days, but the rest either refused surgery or had some other issue that left their gallbladder intact. Seventy percent of those did well without the surgery and needed no admissions to a hospital for the next four years.

Although the procedure has been a boon for many, there are definite risks. When genuinely symptomatic patients get operated on, ten percent get no relief. There is a one to two percent chance of damaging biliary ducts during surgery, which can lead to short term, chronic, or even life-threatening conditions.

If a patient has stones found on a scan and few or no symptoms, shunning surgeons is safest. Stephen Barrett of *Quackwatch.com* summed it up back in 1998 on his list of need-less surgeries. His words still ring true today:

Avoid gallbladder surgery unless you've had at least one severe attack or several less painful attacks in the upper right part of the abdomen, or if you develop jaundice or pancreatic inflammation and tests confirm that stones are the actual culprit. Surgeons should not operate to treat vague symptoms such as flatulence or bloating, which many people—and some doctors—mistakenly attribute to gallstones.

Carotid endarterectomy is the surgical removal of cholesterol deposits from the inside of the carotid artery where it branches before entering the brain. It is an attempt to prevent one type of stroke, where the material breaks free, enters the brain, plugs a smaller artery, and produces brain death or dysfunction. But studies show the surgery helps only for those who have both extensive blockage and a history of prior stroke. If done for people who have not had a stroke, or with less than 50-70 percent obstruction, the patient has more chance of being harmed than helped. The surgeons split a lot of hairs over the exact indications for this surgery.

In a patient with cholesterol deposits, the entire arterial system typically has them and not just the carotid area. These other arteries can cause identical problems. This makes endarterectomy surgery futile for many (possibly most) cases. The procedure itself causes a stroke in at least 5 to 6 percent of operations. Some studies say this number is 20 percent. One patient in 200 dies because of the procedure.

Vascular surgeons often minimize these hazards when counseling patients. They also sometimes operate on people who have not had a stroke and are unlikely to benefit. In the US, surgeons did 140,000 carotid endarterectomies in 2009. They cost $15,000 each. The total is more than $2 billion a year.

In the US, the following are some of the most commonly performed major surgical procedures for rough comparison. The numbers below are yearly totals from several sources.

1) Cesarean section—1,272,000
2) Circumcision—1,108,000
3) Hernia repair—1,000,000
4) Arthroplasty of the knee—728,000
5) Hysterectomy—600,000
6) Angioplasty and stents—560,000
7) Laminectomy (spinal disc removal)—525,000
8) Spinal fusion—488,000
9) Cholecystectomy—300,000

There are grave questions about seven of these nine procedures, given their frequency. Even circumcision has vocal detractors. No surgery is risk free, even if the indications are proper. The financial rewards for providers *doing things* have led to overuse, corrupt practice, and then patient harm.

CHAPTER 27

SCREENING TESTS ARE
USELESS

*The system is not failing. It's functioning exactly as designed. It's
designed to run up health-care costs. It's about the greedy serving
the gluttonous.*

— Otis Brawley, MD, chief of the American
Cancer Society until 2018

We have become obsessed with our medical misadventures.
Every American coffee shop is filled with people chatting
about their doctors, the fees, or their friend's nursing care.
They worry about hundreds of heavily marketed illnesses
and pseudo-illnesses.

Numbers haunt us—cholesterol, bone density, and blood
pressure—as if they were life and death. Entrepreneurial radiologists check carotid arteries with machines set up in shopping malls. Women under 30, whose chances of breast cancer
are almost nonexistent, worry incessantly about it. The
national focus has turned to how sick we all are.

Medical testing was traditionally, and reasonably, used to
clarify what was happening *after a patient developed a symptom*.
Now, however, many tests are used just for screening. This is

an attempt to diagnose conditions *before they happen*, hoping to prevent them. Although it sounds reasonable, the math proves that screening is ineffective and somewhat hazardous. It does churn a lot of healthcare money, however. Look at the stories below and think about which corporation or group profits.

As explained in the previous chapter, suppose a screening test or prophylactic drug like a statin cuts the chances of dying from a particular disease in half. This is a 50 percent improvement in *relative* risk. It sounds great, and researchers use numbers like these to promote findings.

Suppose also that this disease accounts for only two percent of a patient's chances of dying from all causes, the *absolute* risk. This theoretical test improves the *overall or absolute* survival chances by only one percent (.5 x .02). A small number like this disappears into statistical noise. It is of no benefit.

After you understand this, you see that many commonly used routines for healthy patients are an obvious waste of time and money. This includes most colonoscopy, mammograms, cholesterol medicines, and even checking the stool for blood. All these spawn more useless, expensive, and somewhat hazardous medical activities.

Although scientific support for screening healthy patients is lacking, the United States Preventive Services Task Force (USPSTF) produces recommendations for every testing issue. They use committees of primary care physicians and epidemiologists to cook up standards and then vote on them. Sometimes their decisions are sensible. To their credit, they initially said PSA screening for prostate cancer was not worth it. Later, however, when urology concocted the "shared decision making" idea, they approved it, likely because of peer-pressure.

For other cancers, Vinay Prasad wrote, "Why Cancer Screening Has Never Been Shown to 'Save Lives" (*BMJ*, 2016).

He notes that all claims that treatments work are based on relative or disease-specific improvement in mortality, but that improvement of absolute or all-cause mortality has never been shown for any malignancy.

John Ioannidis, according to the *Atlantic* "one of the most influential scientists alive," examined nineteen recommendations by the USPSTF for pap smears, PSA, mammograms, sigmoidoscopy, and others, and concluded they were failures. Like Prasad, he noted that although some of these tests slightly improved disease-specific mortality (relative risk), he found that improvements in overall mortality (absolute risk) were "very rare or nonexistent."

Screening has no benefit for people over 75 years old. This should be obvious even to the worst students of doctor-math. These seniors have a limited time on earth. At that age we all have several conditions brewing at various speeds somewhere in our bodies. It is pointless to try to weed one out and then succumb to something else.

Cancer screening has never been shown to save lives of these elders. For example, the American Cancer Society, even though it has hefty corporate funding, does not sanction routine colonoscopy for this group (2018). Even treatments for a known condition may not affect the absolute risk of death for those over 75 years old. Plying older people with medical technology borders on assault.

PROSTATE CANCER

Urology's approach to this disease has undergone an embarrassing outing. The specialty traditionally recommends that the surgeon draw blood for prostate-specific antigen (PSA). The urologists also insert their finger into the patient's rectum to feel for prostate lumps.

If the blood test is high, or the surgeon feels nodules, they stick a large needle repeatedly through the rectum into the prostate to get tissue samples. If the biopsy shows cancer, urologists recommend perilous surgeries or other alarming therapies. This is all discredited because survival rates never improved for early disease.

The cancer is present but inactive in most men over 50. Ignoring it in the early stages produces the same survival rate as treatment, but without the horrific surgical complications. The commonly performed operation, a radical prostatectomy, produces a 1/200 chance of death. Compromised or ruined sexuality and uncontrollable urination requiring diapers is common, often for the rest of a man's life.

Some patients already have metastatic cancer before surgery. In these cases, it kills the patient even though he has suffered through the grisly procedure and recovery.

The PSA test is unreliable. It increases with any irritation of the gland due to factors such as infection or even bicycle-riding. Antibiotics or anti-inflammatories are the treatments, not surgery. The vast majority of these tumors grow so slowly that death occurs from something else before the disease becomes an issue. PSA is little help to identify aggressive cancers that would be fatal.

Here is a little math: The USPSTF did a large-scale analysis of the research literature. They concluded that for every 1,000 men ages 55 to 69 who had their PSA checked every one to four years for a decade, it would save one man from prostate cancer. The number needed to test is 1000, over 10,000 patient-years, and who knows how many tests, possibly 50,000.

Even if you believe that small numbers like these mean something, the cost-benefit ratio is terrible. False positive PSAs lead to biopsies, which have complications just like the true positives. Men with biopsies that show cancer get surgery or other treatments. The harm resulting from these interventions include erectile dysfunction, urinary incontinence, serious cardiovascular events, deep vein thrombosis, pulmonary embolism, and occasionally death. Checking PSA in asymptomatic men produces no improvement in survival.

The American Veterans Administration "PIVOT" trial compared surgery versus observation for localized prostate cancer over 13 years. There was no statistically or clinically significant difference in either all-cause (absolute survival) or even disease-specific mortality (relative survival). Prostate removal surgery is a net harm.

A Scandinavian study looked at 695 men with prostate cancer who were divided into two groups. One group had radical prostatectomy surgery, the other "watchful waiting." With the surgery, the men were half as likely to die of the cancer (relative death rate), but their overall death rates from all causes (absolute deaths) at five and ten years were identical to those who did not have the surgery. Other researchers support these results.

By 2013, urologists partially responded to the heckling from the rest of the medical community. Their new guidelines recommended "individualizing" this test using "shared decision making" between the doctors and the patients for ages 55 to 69. To understand how misguided this is, consider Otis Brawley's story of an unfortunate patient who was victimized by this system:

Ralph entered the prostate cancer meat-grinder after he had his PSA drawn in a shopping mall at a free cancer screening event. It was 4.3. He had twelve painful biopsies. Two of them showed a moderate grade cancer in about fifteen (15) percent of each specimen. Ralph read everything he could. He decided on robotic surgery because the advertising said it was "advanced." It left him impotent and incontinent, and he required diapers for the rest of his life. His PSA several months later was .9. It would have been zero if the surgeon had entirely removed his prostate.

He became obsessed with the idea that he still had cancer.

So he went to a radiation oncologist who obligingly treated him. When he began seeing blood in his stools later, his surgeons found a fistula. This is a connection between his urethra (urine tube) and his bowel. It was confirmed when he began passing bowel gas from his penis.

The surgeons treated him by sewing his colon to the front of his abdomen with a "colostomy," which required him to change a bag containing his stool several times a day. They also created a similar passage from his bladder to his belly, a urostomy. He still had both when he died of a severe urinary infection a few years later. He was 72.

The urologists, or at least the male ones, do not seem to understand the math about PSAs. Eighty percent of them, along with half the internal medicine specialists, continue to test their own PSAs. Patients have little chance of under-standing any of this if most physicians do not.

Like other diseases with expensive treatments, the prostate cancer industry has nonprofit "advocacy" groups growing in a dense thicket all around it. These universally promote PSA screening, which starts the cascade of billions of dollars of medical services. One organization, *Us TOO*, is 90 percent funded by the pharmaceutical and device companies who profit from this prostate circus. *Zero*, formerly the National Prostate Cancer Coalition, has funding from Amgen, AstraZeneca, Aventis, Cytogen, Merck, Pharmacia, and Pfizer.

Kimberly-Clark, the maker of Depends incontinence diapers, is another donor. Prostate cancer surgery sells a *lot* of adult diapers for them. Zero and the others claim to be inde-pendent, unbiased grassroots groups that are not beholden to any company.

Shared decision making is an abdication of responsibility. We are losing trust in advisers who cannot advise. Fewer and fewer will shoulder responsibility in this age of lawsuits. *Other People's Money*, a book about finance, explains the issue: "A good lawyer manages our problem; a bad lawyer responds to every issue by asking us what we want to do. When ill, we look for a recommended course of action, not a detailed description of our ailments and a list of references to relevant medical texts. The demand for transparency in finance is a symptom of the breakdown of trust."

I recommend men pretend they do not have a prostate unless they get symptoms. (*Disclaimer*: I am not a prostate specialist. There may be advantages to these treatments that I did not find. Prostate cancer therapy has common themes with the rest of medicine, however. It is complex and there are conflicts of interest. The treatment studies have large numbers, small differences, and outsize claims.)

———

COLON CANCER

Looking for this disease using colonoscopy in people without known symptoms has no credible scientific support. Despite this, we spend billions of dollars on it every year. The risks include bleeding, colonic puncture, and an occasional death.

In private, gastroenterologists refer to colonoscopy as "extracting a $1000 bill from the bowel." Wide variations in regional frequency of colon scoping are evidence of overuse. There are standard recommended intervals for repeating the procedure, but some doctors tell their patients to come back for another look more frequently.

In 2018, the American Cancer Society (ACS) reduced the age recommendation for screening colonoscopies from 50 to 45 years old, bringing in millions of extra patients. Most other countries have better control over their physicians. Standard guidelines abroad are to do a colonoscopy only if there is pain, blood in the stool, or other clinical finding.

"Polyp snaring" is the removal of nipple-like fleshy lumps sticking out of the inside of the bowel using wire loops. Since these can sometimes be precancerous, taking them out could theoretically decrease the chances of invasive cancer developing later. The money made from turning this trick is often half a gastroenterologist's income. But with it comes temptations. An anonymous GI lab nurse working in a respected Los Angeles hospital told me:

> **About half the docs here are crooks.** *With every single colonoscopy, they suck a little piece of normal bowel wall into the scope, snip off the healthy tissue, and send it to the lab. They call it a polyp and bill thousands. Since the pathologists get paid just to look at the specimen, they always say the tissue is "non-specific dysplasia" instead of normal. This qualifies as a polyp, at least for billing. These GIs are one-trick ponies when it comes to making money. Colon scoping and polypectomy is all they have besides the occasional ERCP (endoscopic retrograde cholangio-pancreatography), which is a lot harder and more dangerous for the patient.*

We now have Cologuard, a $600 Medicare-reimbursed stool test for colon cancer. This pricing is typical—it is as high as the company can get away with. Compared with colonoscopy, which costs over $2000 and has risks, this almost seems reasonable. Cologuard supposedly detects 92 percent of colon cancers and 42 percent of advanced polyps with every use. The gastroenterologist does a colonoscopy if the test is positive. If they find anything, surgery or endoscopic removal is done.

DO MAMMOGRAMS SAVE LIVES?

This is a politically correct feminist issue that consumes untold time and money. An extensive Cochrane review concluded that this testing does not improve breast cancer survival. This view is supported by others[1].

Recently, independent panels in both France and Switzerland recommended abolishing their recommendations for screening mammography. The Swiss are eliminating their program. No study has ever shown a decrease in overall (absolute) deaths with the use of mammograms.

A *JAMA* study showed an increased discovery of breast cancers using mammograms, but no change in total deaths, which is the absolute risk. They said, "These findings suggest widespread overdiagnosis." For all the frenzied publicity about mammograms, the breast biopsies, the occasional aggressive surgery, and the other treatments, they produce no gain for women.

The following graph[2] shows this. Between 1992 and 2015, there was no consequential decline in breast cancer deaths (lower line). All the money thrown at screening programs has just produced a slight rise in diagnoses (upper line):

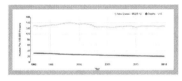

Breast cancer

Even when given the same films over and over, radiologists read mammograms inconsistently. The process does not reveal cancers accurately, nor does it conclusively eliminate the possibility of cancer.

The standard recommendation is to biopsy any suspicious area. This promotes a cycle of diagnostic and therapeutic misadventure. Pathologists look at the specimens, which are often inconclusive. The result is worry, follow-up, and more surgery.

The process is futile with "ductal carcinoma in situ" (DCIS

or intra-ductal carcinoma). A mammogram detects it, then a biopsy makes the diagnosis. The theory is that this is a pre-cancerous or less-invasive breast cancer, so it is treated aggressively. Lump removal with radiation therapy is routine, and sometimes surgeons perform a double mastectomy.

A DCIS study of 120,000 patients undergoing various surgeries and radiation treatments showed few differences in outcomes between the treatments. The authors said: "The choice of... treatment had a strikingly small impact on breast cancer-specific survival, calling for a more thoughtful and restrained treatment approach for this disease." Translated: There was only a little improvement in RELATIVE survival. Since there has never been a study on intra-ductal carcinoma that used a proper (untreated) control group, ABSOLUTE survival improvement is doubtful. It seems likely that not treating the disease at all might have the same ABSOLUTE (all-cause) death rate as treatment.

DCIS appears to be a fake diagnosis (recall, I am not an oncologist). Some studies show that ten years after this condition is found, a patient is slightly more likely to have died from breast cancer but less likely to have died overall. Some suggest calling this finding something other than cancer.

Follow the money. Radiologists profit from mammograms. The surgeons who do the biopsies are wasting resources and taking risks with their patients' health. The congressional committees that support mammograms are grandstanding to further careers.

The charities supporting mammography are in on the action. The United Breast Cancer Foundation and the National Cancer Coalition were among the 50 worst charities in America in one analysis[3]. Over half of the money given to organizations on this list never went for their purported causes. The United Breast Cancer Foundation earned only a two out of four-star grade at charitynavigator.org, which means it underperforms similar charities. The National

Cancer Coalition was worse. They are on the advisory list, which means there is a significant concern for illegal activity, improper conduct, or organizational mismanagement.

Gøtzsche has done an exhaustive analysis of the breast cancer numbers for both a Cochrane review (2013) and his *Mammography Screening* book (2012). He says that screening mammograms and even physician breast exams do not increase survival, and he is outspoken in his opposition to the current approach. He writes that women who discover their own breast lumps are the only ones who should have medical attention.

Note: breast cancer is a real disease. In this chapter, I do not mean to minimize the tragedy for the women stricken by it. My only point is that breast cancer screening for women without symptoms has questionable utility.

CHAPTER 28

FAILED CANCER TREATMENTS

The patient is in the doctor's hands. They will trust you to do
anything at all. You must use good judgment and restraint.

— BILL COOK, MD

CANCER IS MANY DISEASES, and cures are elusive. Slow-
growing tumors rarely require treatment because most never
cause problems and may go away on their own. Fast-growing
tumors are discovered too late to do anything. Only cancers
of intermediate growth rate, a minority, have the potential for
worthwhile intervention.

For most tumors, a modest life extension is the best we can
do. Exceptions include metastatic melanoma, renal cell cancer,
a few lymphomas, leukemias, and testicular cancers. Chemotherapy may extend life or sometimes cure these. Small
numbers prop up the bulk of the other treatments, and careful
analysis shows that the expenses and toxicities may not be
worth it.

Judging what is reasonable in this problematic field
among these relatively weak remedies is challenging.
Communicating the facts honestly and ethically with patients

may be harder. Simultaneously, the physician must manage the emotions surrounding decline and death. This work requires a special person, and most doctors are not strong enough to do it.

Dying patients reach for anything. People with cancer are tremendously vulnerable and have an overwhelming need to trust caregivers. They continue to believe in their doctors, almost regardless of the circumstances.

Oncologists always have new, toxic, and expensive drugs. They may have seen a few patients survive long term using some medication that rarely works and makes everyone sick. They have read studies that showed (maybe) two months' average increased survival with certain drugs. They can usually tell the patient that there is a costly chemo that might help, and it is covered by Medicare or insurance.

It is a demanding job, and the oncologists have a terrific financial conflict of interest that makes it harder. They retail chemotherapy infusions for about a 20 percent markup. Inside the specialty, they call this "buy and bill." By 2013, 65 to 70 percent of oncologists' income was drug charges. Their pay doubled from 1995 to 2004, when it was $335,000, and then it went up again to $445,000 by 2017.

Drug representatives stay in touch with oncologists and let them know whether they are "making their quotas." The companies offer doctors higher percentages for certain drugs if they order more. *This is an inducement to raise the doses of drugs, which can be harmful.* In one egregious case, medications to treat anemia were promoted in this fashion that also increased the chances of premature death. Their sales were $37 billion between 1996 and 2009. Otis Brawley, in *How We Do Harm*, said, "[These] drugs were not used to cure disease or make patients feel better. They were used to make money for doctors and pharmaceutical companies at the expense of patients, insurance companies, and taxpayers."

If two physicians made a deal like this between themselves,

prosecutors might throw them in prison. "Fee-splitting" is a similar, perhaps nearly identical crime where a physician kicks back a commission to another doctor for a patient referral. Federal Stark laws applying to Medicare and Medicaid plus many state laws impose criminal penalties for this. (Between lawyers, however, referral fees are accepted practice.)

Regardless of the exact legalities, our primary priority must be our patients, always. These harmful and unethical incentives draw us away from this duty and must be made illegal if they are not already.

New chemotherapy medications can be 300 times (not 300 percent) more expensive than old ones. Cancer treatment expenses per patient are often over $100,000 a year. Jerome Kassirer adds:

> *One oncologist half-jokingly told me, "Chemo is our cardiac cath, or our arthroscopy,"* implying that chemo offers a profitable *"procedure" for the oncologist [which is] "the dirty little secret of oncology." ...Some oncologists... make an income of nearly a million dollars a year by pushing chemotherapy... approximately two-thirds of the income of oncologists in community practice was derived from intravenous or intramuscular drugs... [Quoting Dr. Eisenberg] "the financial conflicts I have identified in our discipline... are so pervasive and insidious that we continually must remind ourselves as to the real purpose of our work."*
>
> — ON THE TAKE: HOW MEDICINE'S COMPLICITY WITH
> BIG BUSINESS CAN ENDANGER YOUR HEALTH (2004)

Gleevac, for example, is effective for some leukemias but costs nearly $9,000 for ninety 100 mg tablets. In 2014, we spent $92 billion on US cancer therapies, but in 2020, costs are projected to be $173 billion. Some treatments are hundreds of thousands of dollars a year for each person. Even patients who are near death get them. They experience the grim side effects for no benefit.

Only a scant few of the expensive, toxic cancer therapies improve lifespan. Once tumor spread has occurred, most chemotherapy barely helps. Nortin Hadler wrote that survival has been extended only a few months for the most common tumors:

> *Lung cancers (except small cell):* 2-6 months after several chemotherapies.
>
> *Breast cancers:* drugs have not improved survival time. Early diagnosis has increased the number of cases, but death rates have changed little.
>
> *Colon cancers:* from 9 to 22 months for the newest drugs.
>
> *Prostate cancers:* 2 months.

Rethinking Aging (2011)

He said this was another "dirty little secret" that oncologists withhold from the public. There are new drugs every year. Many do not even improve the quality of life.

Dr. Hadler's opinions are dated, but Vinay Prasad, MD, evaluated the cancer drugs approved in 2016-2017. He wrote that they did not extend survival at all. He also studied oncology drugs that the FDA approved between 2008 and 2012. Thirty-six of the 54 were approved using surrogate endpoints and had no known effect on survival. Four years later, only five of them had been shown to help anyone live even a day longer. Prasad's conclusion was that post-marketing studies should be required.

The American Society of Clinical Oncology knows all of this. Their 2014 goal for chemotherapy life extension was only 2.5 months. The 72 cancer therapies approved from 2002 to 2014 resulted in an average of only 2.1 more months of life than the older drugs. Only one in five from 2014 to 2016 worked even that well.

Otis Brawley, MD agrees. He wrote: "I'm starting to hear more and more that we are better than I think we really are. We're starting to believe our own bullshit."

He said specialties that make money on diseases should not be deciding what is reasonable for testing or therapy. For example, radiologists should not be on panels deciding about the use of mammograms, and urologists should not determine radical prostatectomy standards. As obvious as this sounds, it is a radical idea for doctors.

Cancer ads make exaggerated claims about treatments that barely work. Although many of these therapies do not help people live longer, TV commercials typically promise "a chance for longer life."

Dr. Prasad reviewed contemporary news stories for words like miracle, breakthrough, game-changer, and cure. Fifty percent of the time, they were used to describe drugs not approved by the FDA, and 14 percent of the time, they were talking about drugs that had only been tried in mice.

Timothy Turnham, former director of the Melanoma Research Foundation, an advocacy group, said, "there is a disconnect between what researchers think is statistically significant and what is significant for patients. Patients hear 'progress,' and they think that means they're going to be cured." He was referring to chemotherapy approved for surrogate outcomes—a reduction of tumor size or some other result not affecting longevity.

Ad spending for cancer treatments has doubled in the five years ending in 2018. The total spent by cancer centers was $54 million in 2005 and $173 million by 2014. One group, Cancer Treatment Centers of America, did 60% of all the US cancer marketing that year.

Another strategy is to frighten the public by telling them cancers are increasing. Most times, however, the fatality rate, which is the best measure of any cancer's actual occurrence, has been unchanged for decades. Thyroid cancer, for example, is being discovered much more often, as seen in the top line of the graph below, but there is no change in the death rate since 1992, which is the lower line[1]:

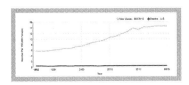

Thyroid cancer

One explanation could be that we are curing more cancers and saving more lives, but this is impossible—most of our treatments are ineffective or barely effective. These diseases are being discovered earlier and earlier by aggressive screening, which accounts for the increase in numbers. We promote anxiety, and we sell drugs. Most of the newly discovered tumors would go nowhere, even without treatment.

In South Korea, ultrasonic screening diagnosed 15,000 people with thyroid cancer, resulting in thousands of radical thyroidectomies, all of which required lifelong thyroid hormone replacement. The surgery caused vocal cord damage in two percent. However, mortality rates were rock-stable. This is proof that this early diagnosis had no benefit and harmed some[2].

Kidney cancer shows a similar pattern. Increases in diagnosis (top line) make the incidence seem to rise, but this has helped no patients. The cancer deaths (lower line) are the same year over year from 1992 to 2014[3].

Kidney cancer

Ineffective or barely effective cancer treatments are costing us a fortune. In 2014, US spending on oncology was $88 billion, and patients spent another $4 billion. Other estimates are closer to $100 billion now. The newest medications, often offering only a few months of progression-free survival, and not extending life at all, cost an average of $171,000 a year (2016). Some are $100,000 a dose. As I published this book, the prices were still higher. They seem to reflect an attitude of "grab what you can."

The industry mantra is that the newest is best, problems are a thing of the past, and that we must trust modern therapies. However, physician experience with many decades of new drugs debunks this. It takes years and thousands of patients before a medication can be deemed reliable. The most likely outcome with any novel treatment is failure or newly found toxicity.

For example, the FDA approved a novel chemotherapy, the heavily hyped chimeric antigen receptor T-cell therapy. This uses genetically modified T white blood cells to kill cancer. The first drug in this class was approved in 2017, so long-term patient survival is unclear. It is mainly used for blood cancers, it sometimes has neurological side effects, and it may only work once. Then the tumors recur. One estimate of the costs, including hospitalizations, is $1.5 million per patient.

Chemotherapy causes fatalities and dementia. For example, Avastin may produce a few months of survival advantage, or possibly the surrogate outcome of a few more months of disease-free survival. Unfortunately, when combined with certain other chemotherapy agents, it may make breast cancer patients die sooner. The FDA carelessly allowed it to be marketed for breast cancer in 2008, but three years later, follow-up studies showed heart attacks, bleeding episodes, and high blood pressure. The agency took the rare step of recalling it.

Even if patients survive, post-chemotherapy mental impairment or "chemo brain" affects 30 percent of everyone treated. This can include memory loss, visual changes, and even brain shrinkage. Tamoxifen, the anti-estrogen drug used for breast cancer, also causes mental impairment. Estrogen is a vital support for many human systems. Women need it to function at their best, and it is important for men also.

THE SKIN CANCER CHARADE

I tried to become a dermatologist once. These specialists stay cleverly in their own world, avoid dealing with serious problems, and make a lot of money without losing sleep. It seemed like a masterful concept. I was an annoying young man, but through family connections and somehow conjuring a fragile veneer of charm, I got accepted into one of their most selective training programs. I thought this feat qualified me for the dermatologic lifestyle and wanted to spend my week-ends hiking the Appalachian Trail. My mentors, however, thought I should spend 70 hours a week learning skin disease. After a year, they exposed me as a poseur and kicked me out.

I viewed it as a personal failure, but the whole time, I smelled something fishy. I was too close to see clearly and I had plenty of problems, so I could not put my finger on it. Like the dermatologists who were unsuccessfully trying to train me, I did not know the history.

The modern era for skin doctors started in the 1980s

when the American Academy of Dermatology hatched a plan to contrive an epidemic of dangerous skin cancers. A Madison Avenue public relations firm charged them two million dollars to come up with the idea. The proposal was for them to disease-monger themselves from foolish pimple poppers into fierce cancer fighters. After this, they evangelized about patients coming to their offices to get a complete skin examination. This would supposedly prevent a plague of skin cancers. The USPSTF later exposed this idea as worthless and said the screening frenzy was cultivating lucrative skin surgery rather than preventing cancer.

One ploy involved proclaiming the skin bumps they call actinic keratoses or AKs precancerous (dermatologists love names and acronyms). Many seniors have dozens, if not hundreds of these. Since then, armies of skin doctors have been billing Medicare for treating millions of AKs with liquid nitrogen devices resembling tiny blow-torches. Studies show that over half of all these bumps disappear on their own. Only one percent change to skin cancer after a year and four percent after four years, and these are virtually all slow-growing and easily treatable.

At about the same time, to handle this pandemic, dermatologists dreamed up the most expensive skin procedure ever seen, "Mohs" surgery. Many of these specialists bill Medicare hundreds of thousands of dollars a year for this alone. I have an acquaintance who does ten of these cases every Friday and gets paid about $15,000 each.

Patients spend up to a full day sitting around an accredited surgicenter operating room while dermatologists remove slices of their tumor bit by bit. They examine each morsel under the microscope as it comes off. A bill is submitted for each cut. There is another for processing each bit into a slide, and yet another for each look into the microscope. This goes on until they have removed all diseased tissue.

After this, the area is "reconstructed." This involves a lot of sewing, sometimes in areas as small as a dime. Insurance pays more if this is performed on a separate day, so the patient often gets sent home with a hole in their face. Sometimes the patients get referred to plastic surgeons, who may use surgical center charges and other tricks to make even more money. In return, the plastics try to dig up skin cancer cases to send to dermatologists for Mohs treatment. These get bounced back to them for reconstruction.

At first, dermatologists did Mohs only for selected patients using careful criteria. Some areas of the body are critical for function and appearance, and their preservation can be essential. For example, this procedure produces excellent results for skin cancers of the nose and corners of the eyes. Other tumors have an octopus-like spread with indistinct borders. Here, Mohs is used to remove just the tumor with as little normal tissue as possible. These issues have all been worked out by dermatologists and published in their journals.

The older methods involved scratching, burning, or cutting away skin cancers. The holes were often left to heal without stitches, and we would then follow the patient for recurrence. With the use of a greasy antibiotic ointment a few times a day, normal healing regenerates the skin within a few weeks. The results are typically reasonable, even on the face.

Although this is adequate for the vast majority of skin cancers, dermatologists now perform Mohs indiscriminately. Robert Stern, a Harvard dermatologist, said, "The decision to utilize [Mohs] is likely to reflect the economic advantage to the provider rather than a substantial clinical advantage for the patient." He reported wide variations in usage by the practice and region and estimated that the costs of Mohs surgery in the US were $2 billion in 2012. A panel charged with developing reimbursement criteria produced vague guidelines that are used to justify almost anything. The experts who were making money made the rule—that they could do nearly anything they wanted.

Mohs is primarily used to remove basal cell or squamous cell skin cancers, which rarely leapfrog to other areas of the body. It is not appropriate for melanomas, which surgeons remove along with a sizable chunk of surrounding tissue to prevent these metastases. Mohs primary advantage is that it reduces the chances of having to perform a second procedure for local recurrence. It also allows the surgeon to leave as much healthy tissue as possible.

The older, much less expensive method is to have the patient return a few months after cutting the skin cancer out to be sure there was no regrowth. This follow-up check takes only a few moments if no further work is necessary. Subsequent removal procedures are usually easy.

Mohs surgeries are medically minor procedures that require only local anesthesia. But the fees are often higher than those for complex, lengthy, and hazardous general surgeries. Dermatologists spend money on lobbyists, who do their job defending exorbitant reimbursement for skin procedures.

Melanoma is the only skin cancer that routinely metastasizes and kills people. The dermatologists almost universally refer these cases to plastic surgeons for removal and then to oncologists for chemotherapy. Few skin doctors want to get involved with a fatal disease.

But when the dermatologists became cancer slayers, they began crying about the exploding numbers of melanomas along with the other skin tumors. As a result, they discovered so many that they made the claim that melanomas were increasing faster than any other cancer. This epidemic now seems to be on the point of slaughtering anyone who dares to walk outside in sunlight.

Left unsaid was that small, early tumors require only a simple procedure rather than an overpriced, supposedly complicated plastic surgery. Treating low-grade (thin) melanomas in seniors does not prolong their lives, either. However, once discovered, since progression into a fatal disease is unpredictable, they are cut off.

Because of all this, far more melanomas are being identified, but the total deaths are not increasing. Like thyroid and kidney cancer, the disease-specific mortality for melanoma has not gone up one iota. All the extra procedures to chase them, however, cost us time, pain, money, and anxiety.

The top line on the graph below is the number of tumors being found. The lower line is the number of deaths, which are unchanged (National Cancer Institute).

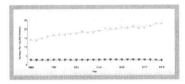

Melanoma

A generous observer might say that the above analysis has not entered the dermatologic consciousness and that there are no wrongdoings here. But the specialty's ringleaders understand it—they orchestrated the entire thing. And they made the story terrifying through disease-mongering.

People over 85 years old get twenty percent of all Mohs surgery. Many get performed in the last year of life, and even in the last weeks before death. Demented people in nursing homes get frozen, biopsied, and operated on. These procedures hurt.

The skin doctors even got approval for a code to bill insurance for pimple-popping or "acne surgery." During my training, when I reached a certain stage, they slapped the specially designed pimple extractor into my hand. I felt like a general surgery resident who was finally being given the scalpel to do my first appendectomy[4].

———

CANCER TREATMENT CONCLUSION

Honest physicians place their patients' interests ahead of their own. This is not always happening for cancer treatment. To an outsider like me, much of oncology seems like a toxic, expensive failure. Some of these treatments prey on people during their defenseless time at the end of their lives. But some work, some are cures, and a few are miracles. You have to do your research, make your decisions, take your chances, and stay hopeful. This field may be changing more rapidly than any other, and some of the outrageously expensive new drugs work.

Dermatologists self-promote and disease-monger. Most of the diseases they handle are cosmetic or nearly cosmetic.

Just like the others, both these specialties cannot resist reaching for all the insurance money stacked around them.

CHAPTER 29

FUTILE CPR AND
OVERPRESCRIBING

Advanced cardiac life support (ACLS) and cardiopul-
monary resuscitation (CPR) are practically worthless. These
are the routines we see on TV in the emergency room when a
patient's heart or breathing stops. Doctor-actors thump on the
patients' chests, blow into their lungs, give lots of drugs, and
dramatically shock their hearts.

On TV, this works. In real life, it consistently fails, except
rarely, when a shock resets the heart's electrical system.
Pushing on the chest helps a tiny number of people, but ribs
get broken all the time. Rescue breathing sometimes works
for pediatrics, opioid overdoses, and a few other cases. The
medications never help.

The training manuals confirm this. One reports: "No
medication has been found associated in any trial with
increased survival to (hospital) discharge." Stated more
precisely: the drugs are proven failures after studying tens of
thousands of patients for decades.

The manual also says: "There was no difference in
outcome between CPR with ventilation and CPR without
ventilation [for adults]." In plain English, rescue breathing is
also useless. The vast majority of patients abused by this

routine are older people whose bodies have failed. There is no chance of success.

The same source, however, quotes the American Heart Association (AHA) standards for the use of injectable adrenaline and CPR breathing. The manual reminds the reader that the AHA require medical providers treating cardiac arrest to use both. The ACLS training manual references are worth citing even though they are behind paywalls, because they reflect the American Heart Association party line. When these ACLS instructors say that their field is questionable, they are credible.

An outsider can google to their heart's content and never be sure about this subject. There is jargon, controversy, and hundreds of confusing references. For example, one of the worst faux endpoints is survival to hospital admission but not to hospital discharge. Who cares, and why would they write this up?

The insiders understand that this system is nearly meritless. The vast majority would refuse CPR and ALCS for themselves. During my residency four decades ago, we each said that we would have *DO NOT RESUSCITATE* tattooed on our chest. It was apparent then, long before the proof developed, that it was a costly, savage, and useless abuse of dying patients.

Becoming ACLS certified entails memorizing and practicing complex, changing protocols. If doctors deviate from these arbitrary rules, we can get sued, and the medical board might compromise our medical licenses.

Emergency physicians have been saying ACLS was bogus for decades, but no-one listens to them, ever, except a few anesthesiologists, who do get it[1].

Out of the hospital, however, simple CPR is worth trying because it occasionally works. A 2010 study of 95,000 patients given CPR on the street in Japan showed that three (3) percent of those treated survived to lead a mostly normal life. The rest died or had brain damage.

Aside by Abe Katz, MD: *This is all accurate, but I can say none of it in public. Remarkably, they force us to perform this charade every day in the hospital, even on COVID patients, where risks to staff are substantial. If we question it, they would label us crazy. Almost every emergency physician understands this, but we have to keep our mouths shut to keep our jobs.*

The colossal American Heart Association (AHA) is the economic driver behind ACLS. Just to train people to perform ACLS and CPR, it pulls in $138 million a year.

The AHA emphasizes their individual donor support on their "meet our donor's" website page. *CharityNavigator.com* likes them. But by 2017-2018, they were spending $887 million a year, nearly 9/10ths of a billion dollars. This has the overwhelming smell of corporate money. If they can avoid industry funding and still generate a budget like this, they are the first group I ever saw to pull it off.

Barbara Roberts, MD, and Martha Rosenberg, in a 2013 Huff Post article, said that, in 2011-2012, $521 million of the AHA's $645 million revenue came from the drug companies and other healthcare corporations. Other sources are also sure that industry overwhelmingly funds this nonprofit.

To be fair to the AHA—which is difficult for me, knowing what I know about them—I had trouble being sure who donated what from reading their financial statements. Detail is lacking, and in 2017-2018, they claimed only about 20 percent of their budget came from corporations. Their pie chart was a blank wedge for the remaining 80 percent. They claimed this was from non-corporate revenue sources.

However, if influence theory is correct, donations of even 20 percent of their budget has strings attached—or more accurately, steel cables. If influence theory is true, commercial interests entirely dictate the AHA's agendas. If influence theory is true, it is a creature, virtually a subsidiary, of the corporations.

Their behavior reflects this. They promote the statins and various big food agendas. They also endorse clot-dissolving drugs for strokes in their cardiac resuscitation training. This is not part of their mission to save the world from heart disease —but they get a lot of money from the drug manufacturers, so they slip it in.

———

OVERPRESCRIBING

Although antibiotics cause harm, doctors hand them out like party favors. Outpatient infections are mostly viral and do not respond. A *NEJM* study published in 2019, "Inappropriate Antibiotic Prescribing in the U.S.," looked at 19 million antibiotic prescriptions. Over half were inappropriate.

When patients' throats are sore, they get concerned. Antibiotics shorten pain by only an average of 16 hours. The medical reason we treat is to prevent rheumatic fever (RF), which can damage the heart, the brain, and the joints. But a million people need to take antibiotics to prevent one RF case, and this causes a lot of diarrhea, skin rashes, and women's yeast infections.

Worse, one in 400 people treated has a severe reaction. David Newman says ten percent of people who get one of these "anaphylactic" allergic reactions die. If this is true, one patient in 4000 dies because of drugs given for dubious reasons. Other sources say two percent of these severe reactions are fatal, which still seems like a lot.

The industry promotes expensive, patented antibiotics. Direct-to-consumer ads were 40-50 percent of the $5.2 billion drugmakers spent on marketing in 2016. For the antibiotic Zithromax, they market straight to children using free toys. Physicians either waste their time trying to re-educate patients or give up and write the prescriptions. Like the patients, many must believe the advertising.

Polypharmacy, the use of many medicines at once, is often worse than using no drugs. Interactions occurring between several medications used together are frequent and may be severe. We know little about this because the FDA only requires the makers to study one at a time. Combinations never get formally tested.

One survey of 7,904 people in Swedish nursing homes found that 65 percent were on ten or more medications. The authors thought seventy percent were potentially inappropriate. Eighty-six percent of the patients were on a psychiatric drug. In Los Angeles, nursing home aides that I interviewed say that the use of twenty (20) medications per patient is commonplace.

Doron Garfinkel studied 119 disabled patients in six geriatric nursing departments and a control group of 71 comparable patients. He stopped 332 different drugs that the 119 patients were taking and made no changes in the control group. Forty-five percent of the control group died but only 21 percent of the study group. The emergency hospital admissions were 30 percent in the control group and only 11.8 percent for the study group.

Prescribing guidelines now command physicians. Every symptom or lab abnormality dictates another drug. Getting our elders off these useless, harmful pills is a specialty. There are articles about how to do it.

Here are some last words about overprescribing by a street-wise Registered Nurse: "I don't think most of our elders would tolerate taking ten to twenty powerful patented medications. It would kill them. Fortunately, under most circumstances, Medicare and insurance companies only pay for generics. Many of these are weak or ineffective. This is the only reason doctors cannot poison our grandmothers."

MEDICATION ANECDOTES: LESS IS MORE

Robert is a 72-year-old contractor who had a heart attack and CABG surgery three years ago. He was taking 11 drugs. Despite monthly trips to his cardiologist to adjust everything, he felt worse and worse over the past year. I thought Robert would feel better on fewer medications, and gently suggested the opioid prescription for his back pain belonged in the trash along with his Neurontin, which was being used off-label for the same thing.

I told him he should try taking Tylenol and tolerate minor discomfort. I also advised him to badger his cardiologist to discontinue some of his heart, sugar, and cholesterol drugs and maybe let his blood pressure drift up some.

Robert ignored my suggestions and quit everything immediately (Note: quitting Neurontin cold turkey is a bad idea). Three weeks later, he felt great, and his blood pressure was still acceptable. I told him his cardiologist had something to offer despite his fondness for medications.

Lurline is 87 years old, has diabetes, hypertension, and heart disease. Her doctors direct her to take 12 drugs. Physicians have always recommended that she take ten or more, but she knows better. She was the poison information telephone nurse for Los Angeles when I was an emergency physician in Pasadena, California. Before the Internet, we would call her for advice about patients who were poisoned with exotic substances.

Lurline says, "if I had taken everything doctors gave me, I'd have been dead a long time ago. I take half, and I decide which half." This may not be the best approach, but she must be better off than if she consumed the lot. She does not worry about her blood pressure of 168/101. How can I argue with success? She is still here and still enjoying herself.

CHAPTER 30

BILLING SCAMS & SPECIALTY WARFARE

Dr. David Morrow had a black belt in billing fraud. His plastic surgery practice was in Rancho Mirage, CA, and his specialty was concocting insurance billing for people having cosmetic surgery. We knew he was making money because he could afford ads in the *Palm Springs Life Magazine* that cost up to $80,000 a month.

Morrow billed his nose jobs as deviated septum surgeries, his breast augmentations as "tuberous breast deformities," and his tummy tucks as treatment of umbilical and ventral hernias. He would brazenly sue his patients' employers if their medical insurers refused to pay. His bills were for as much as $700,000 for a single day's work on one person.

When one of Morrow's clients died during surgery, the plaintiff's attorneys saw what was happening and turned him over to federal prosecutors. By 2017, he and his codefendant wife were facing decades in prison for allegations of $80 million of fraudulent billing. After a plea bargain, just before sentencing, they sold their $9.5 million Beverly Hills mansion, wire-transferred the money abroad, jumped bail, and disappeared.

The police caught them in 2019. The *LA Times* headline

was, "Southern California Plastic Surgeon Extradited Two Years After Fleeing With Fake Passports to Israel." He and his wife, both in their 70s, will probably spend the rest of their lives behind bars.

Morrow was a rotten apple, but his billing practices are still common among his colleagues in Los Angeles. We heard about this for decades from our patients. Putting Morrow in prison has not helped—insurance fraud for tummy tucks and nose surgery is still prevalent.

To get paid for breast reduction, surgeons often claim that the patient has back pain because of her breasts. Some surgeons submit preoperative photos of someone else's enormous breasts and write up faked or exaggerated stories. Some make hundreds of thousands of dollars like this each year.

These insurance scams are hard to spot unless a staff member blows the whistle. Few understand what goes on during surgery, and after the skin is closed, it hides the evidence. The doctors typically conspire with their patients, who get the deductible written off, another illegal practice.

Surgicenter owners have a greedy billing gimmick copied from hospitals—facility fees. These are many times greater than the surgeon's charge. This is for time spent in the building rather than for performing the procedure. It is a novel, shameless idea that could only be acceptable when a third party is paying. Hospitals are allowed extortionate charges because they hire powerful lobbyists. Accredited surgical centers somehow got themselves put in the same category. These surgicenter bills of $50,000 or more for a few hours of work get lost in the hospital billing avalanche and the insurance often thoughtlessly pays.

Because of this, for outpatient procedures, the incentive is always to use an accredited surgical facility or a hospital's outpatient department, where surgeons can inflate billing. Knee injections, a 5-minute procedure, cost $100 in the office. In the surgicenter, the charge might be $5000—or more if the biller includes a facility fee. Unneeded ultrasonic or X-ray guidance, and sometimes even anesthesia, may inflate the cost further.

"Out-of-network" billing also bloats charges. Healthcare systems try to protect their patients from excess fees with contracts. But since 2010, many of the hospital-based specialists have left these networks yet are still billing the same patients for cash. They now charge almost anything they can dream up, even for the in-network patients at their hospital.

These include pathologists, anesthesiologists, radiologists, and emergency physicians. Their patients, who they may never have met, can be on the hook for tens of thousands of dollars if the contracted insurance company does not pay it all. The neonatologists recently piled on.

In 2017, over 15 percent of all patients getting hospital care received outrageous bills from these people despite being insured. Out-of-network doctors may be responsible for half of all overdue debts in America. Forty-three million of us now have medical debt clinging to our credit reports, and this was the top reason for US personal bankruptcies in 2019.

Physicians assisting at a surgery sometimes bill $20,000 for doing work that a nurse or surgical technician could have done. An assistant at neurosurgery billed $117,000 for wound closure at the end of the procedure. A shameless plastic surgeon billed $250,000 for a similar situation. At one time, residents sewed wounds like these closed for free. There are many variants of these swindles. For example, some surgeons operate at a friend's center, the owner bills a colossal facility fee, and they split it.

Dermatologists' pay has gotten so high that their specialty has become an industry suitable for purchase by Wall Street. The largest group in the US is Advanced Dermatology and Cosmetic Surgery. It has four million patients, 192 physicians, 124 physician assistants (PAs), and over 180 locations. They received $600 million from Harvest Partners, a

private equity firm, and are actively buying up more dermatology practices.

Their model is to train physician assistants to take over in
locations that have no doctor. One of their PAs said that her
doctors instructed her to freeze up to thirty skin bumps
during each patient visit. She does pricey skin surgery every
chance she gets on nearly every patient, every appointment,
and Medicare pays for it.

I have heard confirmation of this practice from my
patients. Their dermatologists encourage them to return for a
"complete skin exam to check for cancer" every three months,
and anything sticking up gets cut off or frozen. The bills are
stratospheric. Whenever patients complain about the copays,
the doctors write them off.

**Note: Fee-for-service reimbursement, which is piecemeal
pay for our work, is one root of healthcare evil—and not
just for physicians.** It is a terrific problem for hospitals, insurance companies, and other healthcare corporations of any
species. With the money now being thrown around, patients
are no longer anyone's top priority. To cut corruption and
eliminate improper motivations, doctors must go on salary
and better schemes must be used to pay corporations.

Physician readers: please study this issue carefully before
making your final judgment. I hated this idea during my
entire career and came to it with difficulty. I always tried to
do the best for my patients. I realize now that money is an
overwhelming influence and that everyone's judgment is
subjective, including mine. Patient care is invariably compromised by fee-for-service.

———

**SPECIALISTS FIGHT SLEAZY WARS OVER THE
HEALTHCARE LOOT:**

Every medical specialty and subspecialty organization and their
fellow travelers are lobbying Congress furiously to preserve their
particular turf. It's inelegant behavior, if not downright ugly.

— Nortin Hadler *The Citizen Patient* (2013)

The American Society of Anesthesia (ASA) monopolized propofol, an anesthetic medicine. You may remember this drug; the press smeared it when Michael Jackson overdosed on it along with others. The anesthesiologists claimed propofol had safety issues that other doctors could not handle. They persuaded the manufacturer to label the drug to be used solely by themselves and the nurse anesthetists. Steven M. Green, MD, describes how anesthesiologists connived to do this in *Annals of Emergency Medicine.*

Propofol does not have an increased rate of dangerous events compared to other medications. It is unmatched for safety, patient comfort, and convenience, so it is now frequently and legally used off-label by other specialties despite the restriction. A story from a Los Angeles hospital illustrates why this is not good enough.

John was residency-trained to use propofol to re-locate shoulder joints. It relaxes the muscles, is the safest medication, and is pleasant for patients. Using it, he can get a shoulder back in place just minutes after the x-ray.

But the anesthesiologists at John's hospital reserve propofol for themselves, citing the product labeling. So they involved John in a hospital committee fight. In the meantime, the hospital has directed him to use other drugs. These take longer to wear off and require prolonged monitoring by his nurses. His patients get occasional nausea and vomiting, which he never saw with propofol. He worries about the state medical board hassling him, even if he gets permission from the hospital to use the drug.

This medication also relaxes the bowel, a significant

advantage for gastroenterologists (GIs). They created standards for their nurses to use it under supervision. They say that having highly trained anesthesia providers hanging around checking their email during colonoscopies is a waste of money and that their nurses can do the same job—and check their emails—equally well. They point out that the US anesthesia personnel who sedate GI patients cost a billion dollars a year. But they could not get propofol relabeled.

Shirie Leng, an anesthesiologist, agrees with the critics:

> Anesthesia care used to be limited to very sick patients… Now everyone is getting it… Why did we have to send fully trained anesthesiologists [to the colonoscopy unit]? Because the anesthesia lobby has been powerfully persuasive in limiting the use of some drugs to our docs only… [Propofol] is a powerful drug, but its use is not rocket science… It has been used in other developed countries by non-anesthesia personnel for years. Protecting our jobs looks great from our four-bedroom houses in the suburbs, but not so great for the longevity and integrity of the healthcare system.

The ASA spends one to five million dollars a year lobbying Congress. In 2016, they paid their lobbyists to influence 32 separate bills. Since the labeling change, most hospitals, medical boards, and surgical centers have been against the use of propofol by anyone but anesthesia personnel.

The American Society of Plastic Surgeons (ASPRS) tries to monopolize cosmetic surgery, a multi-billion-dollar market. Traditionally, plastic surgeons perform reconstructive surgery to repair defects such as those created by cancer removal procedures. They are also specialists in hand surgery. But the ASPRS now spends millions of dollars a year advertising their members' supposed superiority in cosmetic or beautification surgery. The procedures they claim are theirs include facelifts, breast implants, liposuction, and tummy tucks.

ASPRS began their anticompetitive behavior over 40 years ago when these procedures started becoming lucrative. In 1975, a lawsuit forced them to turn over internal documents to plaintiffs during a libel action. The following is one of them.

> **We can attack [our competitors] openly** and go back to our posture of reporting their breeches [sic] of ethical conduct (based upon our perspective) to various other medical bodies, or even seek legal solutions in the courts... It is basically a war without end... We would maintain the political mask of constant negotiations ... This group should be men who will not give, but not antagonize their opposite number... [The goal is to] obtain a monopolistic control over a segment of the medical field.

The ASPRS website makes claims that plastic surgeons are the only reasonable choice for cosmetic surgery. One of their videos featured a woman who had massive amounts of liquid silicone injected directly into her breasts. She eventually required a double mastectomy. Below the video, it says:

> In this important PSA (public service announcement) from the American Society of Plastic Surgeons, [the patient] explains how silicone injections in her breasts led to cancer and a double mastectomy. [Her] story highlights the importance of finding a qualified board-certified plastic surgeon to perform procedures. Plastic surgery is real surgery. Be safe. Do your homework.

Injecting breasts with silicone is virtually a criminal act, and this message implies that surgeons other than ASPRS members might do it. Jane Petro, MD, described more about these anticompetitive marketing tactics in the *American Journal of Cosmetic Surgery.*

Messages like these from the central organization embolden individual plastic surgeons to make claims of superiority on their websites and parrot them as expert witnesses. Some have referred their competitors' unhappy patients to lawyers and even paid attorneys to file lawsuits. Jack Anderson, MD, was an early victim of this strategy and retaliated by suing the Georgia Society of Plastic Surgeons.

When the American Board of Cosmetic Surgery (ABCS), a rival of the ASPRS, sought formal approval from the Medical Board of California, the California Society of Plastic Surgeons filed an amicus brief opposing it. The plastic surgeons got California to limit the advertising language that the ABCS members could use. The battle continued at California medical board meetings in 2019.

Contrary to these messages, plastic surgery education offers little cosmetic surgery training. The overwhelming number of malpractice claims related to beautification surgery arise from board-certified plastic surgeons. Other specialties developed liposuction and several other cosmetic procedures with little help from the plastics.

Plastic surgeons' repeated drumbeat is that hospitals, where they have political power, are safer than outpatient surgical centers. There are proportionally fewer complications and fatalities in surgical centers, however, and infection rates are much higher in hospitals. Also, hospital-based surgery had three times the lawsuit rate compared with procedures done in surgical centers[1].

The ultimate fighting championship of the specialty groups is the battle for Medicare payment. Representatives from each group go to an American Medical Association conference held three times a year and fight over who gets the money. Brett Coldiron, a dermatology representative, said this process is like "26 sharks in a tank with nothing to eat but each other." Since many insurance companies copy these decisions, the stakes are high.

They base payment on "relative value units," which favor surgery over the use of "cognitive skills" or reasoning. The factors considered include overhead, the time to perform a service, costs of training, and malpractice costs. Doctors argue for more, and the Medicare representatives say that everyone is getting too much. The specialties spend millions of dollars influencing this process and lobbying Congress.

———

SUMMARY

Doctors believe they deserve to make a lot of money. Bills are routinely "up-coded" or exaggerated to reflect more severe conditions than are accurate. This standard practice may be more of a problem than exotic frauds. Each specialty has also developed a secret garden of dishonest coding and billing practices to defend their earnings. The system is almost without oversight and seems designed to promote dishonesty. Each group aggressively defends their "turf" of procedures and practices where they get their income and where they allege unmatchable expertise.

Postscript: billing riddle. Why are cataract surgeries for two eyes done on separate days? Why are patients brought back for a second or third time when the surgeon could perform several minor surgeries during the same operation?

Answer: second surgeries performed on the same day as the first get half pay, and the third surgery may reimburse only a third. Doctors give the patient various excuses for bringing them back: higher infection rate, too much stress all at once, and if a complication happens, it could be a disaster. The doctors may be right about some of this, but give it some thought if you are in the situation.

A Kaiser ophthalmologist did cataract surgery for me on both eyes, all on the same day, in about the same half-hour.

CHAPTER 31

PATIENT TIPS: FINDING A REAL DOCTOR

TRY to eliminate those of us who are stuffed shirts from consideration. You want someone you can relate to. If possible, get referrals from doctors you know well. If you have no personal ties to a physician, their referrals are unreliable and you will have to talk to your friends. Recommendations from hospitals, where political and financial considerations are operating, are of uncertain value.

You want someone who is keeping up, and so age counts. One of my friends is 45 and works with residents and medical students. He told me that many younger physicians already know most of the stories in my book, which is hopeful news. They may recognize their limitations better. For surgeons, I rarely trust anyone under 50 years old. Standing in the operating room for decades is a beating that somehow gives most of us better judgement and manual skills. Newly trained surgeons are less reliable.

You may already have a bond with your current primary care provider. If they have done their job in the past to help you through the system, they are a good bet. Some physicians assistants are fantastic as well.

You may need specialized help because you have a rare,

serious problem. For some conditions, there are only a few places in the country that deliver the best treatment. Research it—podcasts are an easy way to start. If you have insurance, or better yet Medicare, the charges might be no more than your local hospital.

Major academic centers have many incredible people. For example, Stanford and other elite places select from a group of physician trainees whose test scores are in the top few percent. They are a tiny fraction of an already exclusive group. The specialists supervising these young doctors are brilliant as well. Despite this, even at a top center, examine everything carefully and do not give away your trust easily.

Doctors speak with many people who do not challenge them. Most of us appreciate interesting patients who are reading and broadening their knowledge. Despite all our faults, most of us are authentic people with real human relationships. We will rarely be critical of you if you politely refuse some therapy as long as your decision makes sense and it is unlikely to get us sued.

There are areas outside of ordinary medicine that have merit. Stem cells and bio-identical hormone therapy likely qualify. Another example: I have a friend who runs an alternative oncology group in an area of the country where they like "holistic" medicine. These treatments keep people away from harmful conventional practices, which is a benefit. His doctors are careful to refer to conventional ones when they think other solutions are better than theirs.

Every option, however, is a *caveat emptor* situation. Ben Goldacre wrote:

> *Alternative therapists who sell vitamins and homeopathy sugar pills, which perform no better than placebo in fair tests, have no role to play. These business people often like to pretend, with an affectation of outside swagger, that their trade somehow challenges the pharmaceutical industry. In reality, they are cut from the same*

cloth, and simply use cruder versions of the same tricks. Problems in medicine do not mean that homeopathic sugar pills work; just because there are problems with aircraft design, that doesn't mean that magic carpets really fly.

— *BAD PHARMA* (2012)

Traveling to other countries for your care can be cheaper than obtaining it here. The quality may be equivalent, although this is difficult to evaluate in advance. You must learn enough to convince yourself that whatever you are contemplating has an excellent chance of working.

PART VI

HOSPITALS, WORKERS COMP & THE ACA

CHAPTER 32

HOSPITALS ARE SHARKS

Market economists I've spoken with variously refer to hospitals as "sharks" or "spending machines." With few, if any, market forces to effectively curb their behavior, they raise prices as much as they can. Because most hospitals are nonprofit institutions, they have no shareholders to answer to and cannot legally show a "profit;" therefore, they spend excess income on executive compensation and building Zen gardens and marble lobbies.

— Elisabeth Rosenthal, *An American Sickness*
(2017)

Hospitals cause an epidemic of damage. Estimates for preventable deaths a year in US hospitals range from 200,000 to over 400,000. As far back as 1998, a JAMA report estimated there were 100,000 deaths a year from hospital medication blunders alone. These are the tip of an iceberg of error, for most mistakes cause harm rather than death.

These institutions are enormously influential and wealthy. They gobble about a third of US healthcare spending, which is over a trillion dollars a year. Their supporters include doctors, drug companies, and thousands of employees. Local business leaders throw money their way with pricey donation dinners.

Cardiac or other specialty units often make the most for them. Profit margins for some, such as Ohio State, are over 30 percent.

Over 75 percent of all American hospitals, and eight of the ten largest, are nonprofit. Many were initially Catholic charities run by nuns, who worked for free. Now, the nonprofits operate almost identically to the for-profits but are less accountable because they have no shareholders and no analysts watching them. They make money, and they call it an "operating surplus." The nonprofits and the for-profits spend about the same percentage of their revenue for charity, 5 percent or less.

Rather than declare surpluses or pay tax with the money thrown to them, hospital systems typically build, market, buy equipment, and pay their executives bonuses. They also purchase physicians' practices. These instantly become more profitable because insurance collections improve when hospital "facility" billing codes are used. This can double or triple collections.

Some hospitals buy every healthcare facility in an entire region, then jack up the prices using their monopoly power. Insurance carriers are not as effective in negotiating with these institutions because they may be the only choice in the area.

Providence Portland Medical Center in Oregon is one of these groups. Like many others of its ilk, it grew expansively over the past 25 years. Structured as a Catholic nonprofit and founded by nuns in the mid-18th century, the torrent of healthcare dollars pumped it up over the recent decades.

Providence hired professional administrators and gangs of coders to aggressively bill insurance companies. They gobbled up dozens of hospitals and physician practices in several states and became the third-largest such system in the US. By 2013, revenues were $2.6 billion, and they paid the top administrator $3.5 million a year. They continued to advertise that they were sponsored by nuns and that they were a "not for profit Catholic health care ministry."

They bought the Swedish Hospital in Seattle. After this, in 2015 five neurosurgeons at the hospital were billing over $50 million each, and the top one billed $87 million. Despite these rewards, one neurosurgeon whined that their new internal environment was "toxic [and] repressive." Providence also marked up hospital prices, which sparked local outrage.

For most people, getting hospitalized only happens a few times in their lifetimes. The financial negotiations are unfamiliar and one-sided, and the institution may be the only choice in the area. Illness can be acute and life-threatening, leaving no time for patients to evaluate the expense.

Once you pass through the hospital doors, fees pile upon fees. Even if the charges can be found online, they are hard to understand. There may not be a hint about how pricey it all is until discharge.

In theory, the advantage of paying our outrageous premiums is that insurance companies contract with providers to control their greed. To make this work, patients must confine their care to "in-network" hospitals and physicians. There are pitfalls, however. Since hospital radiologists, pathologists, and anesthesiologists are now frequently off-contract or out-of-network, even well-insured patients admitted at contract hospitals may end up being billed for tens of thousands of dollars.

Hospitals have a retail and a wholesale model. Their wholesale prices, which are still profitable, are for Medicare and contracted insurance companies. Although their executives are heard to gripe that Medicare does not pay them well, many use billboards to pull these patients into their system.

Hospitals compute their bills using their "chargemaster," a

list of the highest prices for thousands of services. A Tylenol is $10, a gauze pad is $60, and an alcohol pad $8. Chest X-rays might be $289, but Medicare only pays $32. Blood drawing charges, which Medicare ignores, are often $36.

All this adds up if services are performed daily for weeks. After a month, if you are partly in intensive care and have had a surgery or two, the bill might be nearly a million dollars.

Anyone can get sucked into this system. For example, you are 60 and in good health. You have some chest pain, learn that you have an aortic aneurysm, and need surgery. The procedure plus weeks of hospital care cost a half-million dollars.

Or you have a cough for a few days and suddenly can't breathe. Your doctor diagnoses you with unusual pneumonia. Or you might have a health problem but be out-of-state or out-of-country where you have no coverage. Maybe you are 37 years old, between jobs, have no insurance, and get into a car accident.

Or you are an uninsured kid who gets an unnecessary, unwanted helicopter trip to the emergency room because of a heavily bleeding scalp laceration. You were too shy to turn the ride down, and you owe the full $11,000 because the predatory ambulance services rarely negotiate charges. Or maybe the doctors diagnosed you with cancer, but your insurance only covers $2000 a day for hospital bills. You go to MD Anderson, which is the best, but they want $86,000 to get started on the first two weeks of evaluation and chemotherapy. They make you sit in the lobby for hours until your father's check clears.

You sign up on your employer's website for a health plan that cost $600 a month less than the others. It has only $200,000 maximum coverage, which seems like a lot of money, and you did not give it much thought. But you get hospitalized, and when you get out, your bill is $490,000.

Nobody cares about debt when it is paid by someone else, but being surprised by a statement like this gets personal.

The courts enforce hospitals' rights to charge whatever they want, no matter the circumstances. In each case, if you survive your health problem, you have an obligation that might prevent retirement. You have become a debt-slave if you cannot bankrupt—for example, if you own a house you do not want them to seize. Hospitals frequently grab real estate. Medicare protects patients better than most insurance policies, but you can only get it if you are older or disabled.

Here is how the billing works. Before any medical care (even a biopsy) gets done, the hospital does an investigation of your ability to pay. This "wallet biopsy" uses your social security number.

Later, the chargemaster table of fees is used to contrive exorbitant bills. When interviewed by Steven Brill for his *Time* article, hospital executives were apologetic about this capricious and embarrassingly aggressive practice. Since the prices are pure fiction, no-one inside the industry can explain them.

After they tally the bill, they make adjustments if you have insurance or Medicare. Sometimes, Medicare only "allows" twenty percent of the original charges, and throws out eighty percent, including junk charges like Tylenol and gauze pads. Lab tests often get reduced to less than $10 from hundreds. The hospital prints the last bill and sends it to you.

Those without insurance get charged top dollar. Hospitals view this as the start of a negotiation, but the billing stuns patients. Even if you have insurance coverage, the copays and other fees can be horrific.

Most patients are ill-equipped to understand the process or deal with it, especially when they are ill or recovering. They respect their doctors and other providers and do not expect the hospital to treat them like this. The nonprofit hospitals have a reputation for being particularly ruthless.

Hospitalization is the ultimate seller's market. The patient is in the institution without other choices, and they must purchase hospital CT scans and other services at retail prices. Even if they could compare their complicated options somehow, patients are sleeping in the institution as the bills pile up.

Hospitals bill whatever they want. They have office buildings full of highly trained coders and collection agents. Their job is to get the highest cash, Medicare, or insurance payment by using the most inflated charges and imaginative descriptions they can dream up. If you are uninsured, they go after you voraciously. No-one will protect you.

Hospitals sometimes pay physicians who work there based on their ability to code their services. The institutional billers routinely encourage doctors to up-code or exaggerate, and if they bill less aggressively, it may cost them money.

For example, Dr. Katz is being monitored by his hospital's coder. He was once told, "if you get x-rays and order a pain shot for that back patient in the emergency department, you could justify a level 5 instead of a level 3 charge." They are saying that, rather than use his best judgment, he should order inappropriate studies and therapy to make the hospital more money.

Here is another anecdote. Maria is a patient of mine who called the ambulance 30 minutes after she arrived home from her minor surgery. She had some minimal bleeding, and she is an excitable individual. I called the hospital and told them she was coming and recommended they send her back to my office. The emergency room nurse looked her over and could see the patient was fine.

However, the physician assistant who saw her ordered chest and abdominal x-rays and $800 worth of blood testing. When I spoke to him about it, he reminded me it was all paid by Medi-cal, the California Medicaid program, so it was free for the patient.

On top of other costs, a cottage industry of billing advocates has arisen. They repeatedly call the hospital collections center until they find a person willing to negotiate. They can cut most charges by 30 percent on the phone, but it gets harder after that. The advocates charge about $100 an hour.

Just like other corporations, hospitals aggressively disease-monger. They frequently sponsor free skin examinations, PSA testing, and flu shots. Otis Brawley interviewed a hospital marketer regarding their PSA screening in local shopping malls. He said that they made a lot of money from this. It helped pay for all their other "product lines," including their breast cancer center and chest pain center. He described how it worked. Fifteen percent of the men who get their PSA drawn have an abnormal result and are advised to visit the clinic. Charges for this first evaluation alone paid for all the initial blood tests.

The marketer knew the percentage of these men who had insurance, the revenue from the ensuing biopsies, and the percent whose biopsies showed cancer. He knew the "downstream payments" that the hospital would get for the radical prostatectomies, the radiation, and even the hormone suppression therapy. He also had the numbers of patients who would ultimately need penile implants for impotence, and those who would need an artificial urethral sphincter implanted for incontinence.

When Brawley asked him if he knew whether the process saved lives, he replied, "Don't you know, no-one knows if this stuff saves lives. I can't give you a number on that."

Conclusion: The nonprofit hospitals, which have far less oversight than the for-profits, are some of the most ruthless and grasping businesses in America. Costs of their services have grown faster than any other healthcare sector. We deserve better than a system that encourages these entrepreneurs to prey on us[1].

CHAPTER 33

PATIENT TIPS TO BEAT THE EXPENSE

Avoid the price gouging. First, lower your trust for physicians and the rest of the system. Question everything—preferably before it happens. You need to do your research, speak up confidently, and never be intimidated.

Hospitals negotiate their fees, even after performing the service. Find out what your insurance network delivers, how much the hospital will charge, and how the copay works. Websites such as *clearhealthcosts.com* can help you learn about your purchases, with or without insurance.

Be careful about your choice of institution. Their charges are all different. Hospitals are now required to post their prices online, but they are hard to find. Websites like *Floridahealthpricefinder.com* can help you avoid the worst gougers. You may be limited to only a few hospitals because of where you live, but you likely have some choices. Learn about this before you get sick.

Be *very* careful about what you sign. One of the most detestable things I read was having patients sign a contract when they enter a hospital or emergency room. It typically says you agree to pay *anything they charge*. This is improper, especially when you are sick, and it happens in no other industry.

You or your relatives—no matter how defenseless and ill you feel—must read the fine print and cross this clause out. Under many circumstances, the law requires healthcare facilities to take care of you, anyway. If collections agents call you later, request a copy of this contract. You may never hear from them again.

Consider insurance with limited coverage if you can find it. Your policy is paying for the whole Pandora's box of useless healthcare for everyone. Your premiums continue even if you refuse all care.

Proper limited policies are still unavailable as of this book's publication date, but if this changes, using one could help you control costs. I would get rid of psychiatric coverage first if that were possible. You do not want a limit on total expenditures.

Do your homework before you get sick. My book is an introduction, but I recommend a careful study of Nortin Hadler's work. He says that if the benefit of therapy is questionable, do not risk the harm. Invasive heart procedures for coronary artery disease are one example among many. For more, review Elisabeth Rosenthal's suggestions in *An American Sickness* (2017).

CHAPTER 34

THE SECOND WORST SYSTEM

I DESCRIBE *the worst healthcare delivery structure at the end of this chapter.*

The US workers compensation (WC) system was based on well-meaning ideas, but it has developed into a mess. The original plan from the early twentieth century and before was meant to streamline companies' payment for work-related injuries, avoid delays, and decrease conflict. It was to benefit both the worker and the employer. The system paid for medical expenses and lost wages. Payment schedules codified compensation for various accidents, such as amputations and even death. "Pain and suffering" or "non-economic damages" were not compensable. This simplified a poorly quantifiable area.

Although there are federal guidelines, each state developed a separate undergrowth of laws and idiosyncrasies. In 2017, workers compensation covered 140 million US jobs and 42 percent of the population. About 80 percent of the WC obligations are passed through insurance companies, and the client corporations retain the rest of the risk.

In 2017, employers' costs for workers compensation, according to the National Academy of Social Insurance, were

$97.4 billion, and the benefits paid were $62 billion, which is 64 percent of the total. Insurance company profit, overhead, and administration are the rest—a calamitous 36 percent. Recall that other types of insurance may have total costs of up to 25-30 percent. If this were the only outlay needed to supervise the system, it would about match the rest of healthcare. But there are many others.

A second expense layer is the contingency-fee lawyers. They get involved with 28 percent of cases nationwide and take a percentage of any award. Litigation has derailed the WC system: a study of closed cases from 2007 to 2017 in 46 states from one insurer found:

- Litigation increased claims expenses nearly four times
- Final awards for litigated cases were seven times higher
- Lost work time nearly tripled in lawyer-assisted cases
- Average claim duration with attorneys was 901 days
- Average claim duration without attorneys was 305 days
- California claim duration with attorneys was 1139 days

Attorneys get used more often in the lost time and permanent disability cases, the big ones, so the above effects may not be entirely because of the lawyers.

Frauds are ubiquitous in workers compensation. For the claimants, these include faked or exaggerated claims, off-the-job injury claims (not insured), and claims of disability continuing after actual recovery. The employers also sometimes cheat. For example, they may withhold payments to the insurer in various ways. Doctors may exaggerate or fabricate bills, treatments, or diagnoses. The lawyers may coach them on how to fool the system to get the most money out of it.

Estimates of the fraudulent WC claims for the United States range up to $30 billion a year (2018). This is 48 percent of the $62 billion that made it past the insurance layer. Besides the expense, all that graft creates a climate of distrust, which destroys patient care and breeds more litigation.

A guess at total costs follows. Cut this speculative 48

percent fraud in half and add it to the well-documented overhead consumed by insurance administration, 36 percent.
Combine this with another (conservative) 5 percent spent on
attorneys and litigation. Providers, who have to manage
payment delays lasting two or more years, have billing and
other costs that must be over 10 percent. The total—an
educated guess for the system's expenses—is 75 percent.
Whatever the actual amount is, it departs the system before
care is given to the first patient.

US WORKERS COMPENSATION COST (2017)
US employers' cost for WC in 2013: 97.4 bn
Total US benefits paid by insurance: 62.0 bn 64%
AN EDUCATED GUESS AT THE OVERHEAD:
Expense of ins. co. administration (above): 36%
Rough fraud losses (using lower figure): 24-48%
Estimate of litigation costs (conservative): 5%
Provider overhead costs (conservative): 10%
TOTAL OVERHEAD COULD BE AS HIGH AS 75%

There is worse news: patient outcomes in the workers
compensation system are inferior to those using ordinary
insurance. WC patients take longer on average to return to
their jobs and have more extended disabilities and a higher
percentage of permanent disability.

A senior expert witness, whom I will call Albert, has been
observing the scene in California for 30 years. He says the
insurance industry would rather spend more money on litigation than to recognize disability and fund timely care. Many
cases are held up for years, which can be disastrous for those
with genuine health issues. He says that even though this
delay runs up the ultimate cost of settlement, when the
companies keep the money longer, they make more overall
because they invest the withheld cash and have high returns.

Just like the other players, Albert works the system. He
has forty employees and contractors, and bills the WC insurance companies at his lucrative physician's rate for some

work his employees do. He told me this is a "grey area." His income is $2 million a year, he works 20 hours a week, and he requested anonymity.

These financial gains for lawyers, doctors, and patients divert everyone's focus away from the simple goal of making people well.

Personal injury (PI) lawsuits have their uses, but as a healthcare delivery system, they are disastrous. Here is the basic version of how it works. To start, some injury is necessary. This can be for anything from an auto accident, to medical malpractice, to chronic asbestos exposure. The injured person finds a lawyer, or the lawyer finds them, which is illegal (this is "ambulance chasing"). If there is a wrong or negligence involved with the injury—which means someone is to blame—and they have money or insurance coverage, the attorney sues.

To treat the injury or condition, the lawyers refer patients to doctors specializing in PI. These physicians do their work on a lien, which means they assume all costs and get paid years later when the case gets resolved.

The settlements for PI are traditionally three times the doctors' bill. The doctor gets a third; the attorney gets a third, and the patient-plaintiff gets a third. This encourages physicians to run up their charges to produce a bigger award. Patients may also exaggerate, especially in subjective areas such as emotional injuries. I had coaching about all this from a lawyer when I handled a few personal injury cases early in my career.

In these situations, many physicians charge stunning fees, and they may entirely invent care. A Los Angeles anesthesia provider told me that the orthopedists in his operating room routinely bill $500,000 (a half-million dollars) for a single PI spinal fusion surgery that takes an afternoon to complete. True, they have to fight for their money years later when the bills get negotiated, but this is the starting figure.

Recall that these surgeries have no scientific support. On average, they do not help pain or decrease disability. Some speculate that the operations increase chronicity and long-term pain.

PI has even more fraud than WC. For example, there are many reports of cars full of volunteers, often impoverished migrants, purposefully staging collisions with well-insured commercial truckers. This dangerous scam would never get orchestrated if it did not have substantial financial rewards for everyone involved. The stories about personal injury rackets seem endless.

WC does not function precisely like PI. Still, there is a relationship between settlement size, doctors' charges, lawyers' charges, and the documented extent of the injury. This creates incentives to delay and exaggerate everything. Resources are wasted, fraud multiplies the expenses, and the result is degraded care. It is the same triad as the rest of American medicine: loose money, corruption, and then poor-quality healthcare.

PATIENT TIPS TO BEAT WORKERS COMPENSATION

As you have learned, even for on-the-job injuries, your employer's ordinary health insurance might do the best job with the least down-time and hassle. But enormous posters in the employee lunchroom advise you to "preserve your rights" by filling out all the paperwork and jumping into the claims process.

Despite the problems with workers compensation, putting job-related healthcare issues through the system is unfortunately preferable. There is no limit on coverage, and unlike regular insurance, the company cannot cancel the policy. Providers will always ask you if your issue was work related, and you would have to lie to them if you do not want to go through work comp. Also, insurance companies try to wiggle out of responsibility for anything they can. If they find out later that your problem is a job injury, they may try to reverse the payments.

Despite all this, using the health insurance plan might sometimes save time and hassles. It is also cheaper for the employer. I cannot formally recommend this, and if you do it, be careful. Note also that if you file for workers compensation and get denied, the insurance plan will take care of you.

Providers like Kaiser Permanente use both types of payment, and the treatment is identical. The workers compensation cases pay better, so the Kaiser people will fill out the paperwork for you.

PART VII

CONCLUSIONS AND SOLUTIONS

CHAPTER 35

LEGISLATIVE SAUSAGE-MAKING

The enemy is within the gates; it is with our own luxury, our own folly, our own criminality that we have to contend.

— CICERO

THE FOLLOWING brief history of the Affordable Care Act (ACA) shows how bitterly reform gets resisted by moneyed interests. The drafters tried to improve the American health-care system but mostly failed.

Unlike physicians, the politicians who attempted to repair the system understood the powerful forces opposing them. And, contrary to some accounts, they attempted to cut costs. One special-interest group or another beat back nearly every reasonable idea.

For example, malpractice reform could save billions of dollars. Doctors might be more efficient and order fewer unnecessary tests. This was upended by politically active trial lawyers, who are massive contributors to the Democratic Party. Perversely, these attorneys are considered stakeholders in healthcare, just like patients, physicians, drug makers, device manufacturers, and even insurance companies. The lawyers take a sizable share, sometimes a third, of litigated claims, which is billions of dollars. They can afford lobbyists.

Drafters of the Affordable Care Act made little progress with drug costs. They knew that negotiating drug prices at the federal level could save up to half of our total expenditure (even without uncovering the drugs that do not work). This is tens of billions, possibly hundreds of billions of dollars, every year. Other countries do it, and the pharmaceutical companies still make tons of money.

There were also attempts to change the disastrous 2003 law that prevents Medicare from negotiating their wholesale fees with drug companies. Squashing this was a top corporate priority, so these ideas got nowhere.

The ACA installed a seemingly innocuous rule that allowed pharmaceutical companies to fund out-of-pocket copays for expensive, patented drugs. This is not a charity—it sanctioned a devious practice. When there is no copay, the manufacturers can charge about anything they want because when the patients pay nothing, they care little about costs.

Outrageously priced patented drugs become even cheaper for the patient than generics with this "copay support," because generics force the patient to pay at least a little out-of-pocket. The prices can now increase almost without limit.

The insurance companies care little about total costs because they pass increases on to government or corporate funders and get their piece of the pie, anyway. Arguably, their incentive is to *increase* overall spending.

The ACA drafters also considered allowing the importation of medications from other countries. This would lower drug prices because negotiated costs elsewhere are often half of ours or less. Congress debated and shot down this sensible strategy over and over for the last few decades. Once again, it went nowhere.

The payers gave their input. Craig Barrett, the CEO of Intel, said his company's yearly healthcare expenses approached a billion dollars. As he became progressively more disgusted with the reform process, he was forced to play his last card. Barrett said that healthcare made the US a less competitive place to do business. He was threatening to take part or all of his $62 billion in revenues abroad.

The Affordable Care Act implemented a few excellent ideas. Hospitals could no longer be as abusive with their bill collections. Insurers had to do a better job of explaining what their forms meant. The ACA also mandated an independent appeals process for cases with denied insurance coverage.

Tens of millions more people became insured. The policies could no longer exclude pre-existing conditions from coverage. The law prohibited annual and lifetime payment caps. These three reforms were reasonable and long-overdue, but were a victory for the industry. Healthcare consumption and overall costs both increased.

Jonathan Gruber, who designed Romney's healthcare plan when he ran for president, told the ACA team, "trying to control costs too much dooms whatever you do because the lobbyists will kill you. That's what happened to Hillary in 1993." He said special interests would allow only one type of reform: insurance subsidies, which are customer creation. This happened with the Affordable Care Act. After the corporations negotiated what they wanted, they lobbied alongside the Democrats, and the bill slid through Congress. Universal coverage would also have been acceptable to the industry—it would give them more money.

Despite their core of idealism, the Democratic party had to face reality. There were too many dollars talking for any substantial changes. The reformers could not challenge the insurance companies and their downstream payees, the drug makers, physicians, hospitals, and the rest of it. Steven Brill wrote: the system continued as "substandard care at exorbitant prices" (*America's Bitter Pill*, 2015).

Chapter postscript: During this time, the Obama adminis-

tration and Congress mandated electronic medical records
(EMRs). This was a forward-thinking idea that experts said
was long overdue and would save billions of dollars. The
computer era seemed to dictate this, but it is a disaster.
Doctors now spend the bulk of their time looking at computer
screens and clicking rather than making human eye contact
with patients.

Rather than using Apple to set up a convenient, universal
system, several companies cobbled together competing
schemes that were purposefully designed to avoid integra-
tion. These also facilitated the use of as many billing codes as
possible.

The earliest cost estimates for the software alone were
$15,000-$70,000 per provider—possibly $50 billion or more
total. The investment of doctor time is more costly than this.
Physicians are forced to spend about 16 minutes per patient
messing with the EMR. This is about half their time. They
either do this, or they do not get paid. This effort comes out of
their moments with their families or their duties to patients
and causes burnout.

As an experiment, I obtained a medical record of a two-
week hospital admission. I tried to print it, but I gave up after
I had six inches of paper. It was mainly nursing notes. They,
too, have to click box after box, document bowel movements
and anything else that happens. The substantial events of the
hospitalization were summarized in four typed pages that
were dictated by a physician.

Lawyers now subpoena the entire electronic medical
record, which includes all the provider and nurse clicks. The
whole thing is interpreted retrospectively, as lawyers are
trained to do. This, of course, includes their speculations
about altered records based on mistaken or corrected clicks[1].

As hopeless as all this seems, I present cures that would
work in the next chapter.

CHAPTER 36

SAVE OUR NATION

And I knew there was no victory in this world without another,
larger loss hiding within it, that in our triumph we are already
hunted by some disaster.

— Vikram Chandra, *Sacred Games* (2006)

WE HAVE no choice but to act—we are being cannibalized.
Since the following would shunt money away from the corporations, these ideas will be bitterly resisted.

Remember where we are. Most of US healthcare is
funneled through insurance companies, which burn 20
percent or more of all our industry's spending. Doctors and
hospitals chase the remaining funds. Their administrative
costs are 40.6% and 29.6% respectively. These medical
expense numbers are so byzantine and overwhelming that
guesses about the total are speculative. We have by far the
highest spending and the highest overhead in the world. And
no one ever acknowledges that half our services are useless.

The FDA is impotent. Its budget is only $5 billion, but its
mission is to regulate a fifth of the US economy—four trillion
of the 20 trillion total. This is 800 times larger than the agency.

Worse, the FDA is "gifted" the lion's share of their budget directly from industry, so strings are attached.

Here is what we are dealing with. The healthcare companies are organized, they know what they want, and we permit influence purchasing—lobbying and many other strategies—at every level.

Our fractious nation has no uniform strategy and no cohesive will. Worse, few of us know that corporate racketeers are walking among us. We still believe that providers' top priority is patient care. Billions of dollars are being stolen and our bodies are being damaged. Some of us are dying.

Here is what we must do. Much of healthcare boils down to monster corporations repeatedly settling some of the most massive criminal fraud and payoffs cases in history. Other wrongdoings include disease-mongering, advertising lies, and systematic promotion of scientific misconduct. *Many of these actions are unethical but still legal, so we must define these definitively as crimes and prosecute them aggressively.*

We accept incomplete reporting and hiding data as standard practices. Litigation is the only way to pierce corporate confidentiality rights. But the courtroom reveals only a tiny part of the information, not enough to hold the companies to account.

Medical ethics say that we must share all knowledge for our patients' benefit—honestly, openly, and without charge. Secrecy is misconduct. Medical publications that contain concealments and distortions are unconscionable. *This scientific wrongdoing must be criminalized.* The ridiculously high journal prices preventing scientific exchange would fall as the corporate funding declines.

We must preserve all studies online, both the failures and successes, along with complete data. This begins with registration before studies start, which would ensure that nothing disappears. *Alltrials.net* and *opentrials.net* are efforts to do this, but the companies are resisting. (Síle Lane discusses this in a

Ted talk.) If more comprehensive information were available, we would shame and discredit ghostwriters, their corporate sponsors, and the physicians allowing their names as authors. *Since our public funds pay these companies, we must change the laws so the public, not they, owns all drug and medical product information.*

Doctors involved with corporations must have mandatory recusal from medical standards decisions. *We must prosecute conflicts of interest as criminal acts the same way we do insider dealing in financial markets.*

The US Institute of Medicine and another physician's group, No Free Lunch, call for the elimination of physician gifts from drugmakers. The American Medical Student Association agrees: they refuse to see drug representatives, and their journal refuses their advertising. *Corporate gifts and sponsorship must be defined as bribery and prosecuted.*

Paying doctors, hospitals, and other providers piecemeal bakes in greed, conflicts of interest, and unscrupulous behavior. Billing fraud and exaggeration are now ubiquitous, and we reward unneeded care. What happens to a neurosurgeon who bills $50 million a year? Are they still physicians? Do financial incentives improve patient care, ever? *Fee-for-service must be eliminated.*

Finally, why do we allow corporations to use our public money for healthcare lobbying and medical advertising? We must criminalize this.

———

NOTHING **in this scrum has resembled a real marketplace for decades.** We are long past free-trade solutions. Prices are climbing skyward, which would be paradoxical in a market situation. Those who suggest we can decouple from our collectivist payment systems and go back in time to the halcyon days of the country doctor are unrealistic.

Is our entire government big enough to control healthcare? US spending on medical services is about $3.65 trillion. Our federal tax revenues in 2019 were $3.3 trillion (America borrowed another trillion in 2019 and several more in 2020). *The entire government is about the same size as the healthcare sector.*

Would central control or a single-payer help? Countries that leverage their entire purchasing power to bargain with giant drug corporations pay much less than America does. They are still poisoning their populace, but at least they buy the chemicals wholesale. At the federal level—theoretically— there is also the expertise to avoid frauds and evaluate what we need.

Given Washington's history of incompetence, a single payer could be worse than what exists now. They already run three such groups, Medicare, the Veterans Administration, and the Indian Health Service, all of which are in disarray. During any transition, interest groups would try to grab anything they can. Without proper anti-bribery laws, the same companies would still control the new system.

———

STEVEN BRILL WROTE **that the large hospitals should include insurance in their services.** This would promote evolution toward cost control and proper care. It is a good idea, and we already have a model, Kaiser Permanente. This is the country's largest and oldest health maintenance organization. They integrate their doctors, hospital group, and insurance company into a single system. Each is subordinate to the goal of producing cost-effective, functional healthcare. Simplifying billing and getting the three groups to work together results in huge savings. Physicians are on salary, giving them objectivity that few US practitioners enjoy. Executives are not rewarded for jacking up stock prices.

Kaiser's revenue was $84.5 billion in 2019. They had 12.2 million patients and were growing explosively. That year, they were about the same size as the largest pharmaceutical company, Johnson and Johnson. Their care and management are reasonably well regarded, and they have economies of scale. Workers compensation is integrated. Kaiser has minimized litigation by using arbitration contracts and other oversight. This fends off some lawsuits and resolves others less expensively.

Kaiser is far from perfect, and you must not blindly trust them with your health. They were substandard several decades ago, but have improved. Their nurses and other personnel are unionized, which may make them less responsive. For rare health conditions, you should carefully consider consultation and care outside their system. Although they resist, you can make them pay for it if you are aggressive.

Giving the money to entities like these could bring down costs if funding was based on actuarial healthcare costs per year of life. Money for individual procedures, hospital stay-days, or any other itemized care rewards misuse.

Finally, we must get rid of bad therapies. To start, we can model other countries' more conservative, less wasteful standards. Although many try to copy us, they only squander about half what we spend per person. The goal is to incrementally defund mammograms, angioplasty, CABG surgery, routine colonoscopy, parts of orthopedics, and most of psychiatry. A retired general could take charge of the oncologists and decide about the corporations' chemo drugs. The dermatologists should be transferred to the private sector with the cosmetic surgeons. They could refer for actual diseases.

These changes and the others could save half of our healthcare spending—nearly $2 trillion--without worsening patient outcomes. There will be many arguments, but remember the rule—*if there is controversy, and the numbers are large, the treatments are worthless.*

———

OTHER CRITICAL IDEAS

I initially opposed the following, but I see now that the time for half-measures has passed. The first (✪✪✪) would likely cure the biggest problems in healthcare.

✪✪✪ The abolition of healthcare patents: The twenty-year exclusivity was conceived to encourage research. Sadly, this system made the drug and device manufacturers nearly untouchable. David Healy, MD, and others say that patents must last a few years at most. We would then barely need an FDA[1].

Since half of medical research is government-sponsored anyway, little would be lost if corporations were out of the development game. Company funding for the CDC and the National Institutes of Health must also be forbidden. This would discourage me-too drugs, and ruining data would be more difficult. The pace of industry would slow, and contract research organizations would vanish.

✪✪ Taking most drugs off prescription and making them over-the-counter would start a revolution. Many other countries have partially done this. David Healy says that informed individuals with access to medications over-the-counter make better choices than doctors using prescriptions. I have doubts about this, but our current system is ruinous. We must move to a less paternal and authoritarian system.

If patients were in charge and felt personally responsible, they might not ignore side effects. For example, if a patient taking an antidepressant started feeling terrible, they might quit. They might avoid hanging themselves, shooting school-children, stabbing their wives to death, or throwing themselves in front of trains. Better yet, they might look the drug up on the Internet before taking it, and ignore their doctor's advice.

This is not a cure for the drug marketing plague. Slick

salespeople can sell anything, no matter how useless—
witness what is going on now. In the 1950s and before, huck-
sters sold over-the-counter concoctions using outrageous
claims, but they at least had to compete on price because
there was no insurance. *Healthcare marketing must be criminalized.*

Note this well. Whatever else is decided, we must
continue to restrict opioids and amphetamines tightly, for
they have powerful evil effects. Antibiotics belong in this
class too. The psychiatric drugs should be outed and their
usage monitored as well.

The FDA schedules prescription drugs based on their
abuse potential. The SSRIs and benzodiazepines are both
Schedule IV. The atypical antipsychotics are not abused
because they make people feel terrible, so the FDA does not
schedule them. But all these medications have *addictive* qualities. They should join opioids and amphetamines in the
closely watched FDA Schedule II category of dangerous
drugs. The Tylenol-hydrocodone opioids, Vicodin and the
related drugs, which are now III, should also be switched
to II.

**Deciding on proper care is simple; the politics are diffi-
cult.** Elisabeth Rosenthal recommends committees for establishing medical standards. Shannon Brownlee, another
respected commentator, agrees. In the UK, attempts to do this
are being made. These groups set priorities for limited funds.

But this is like a Noah's Ark, with pairs of animals representing each "stakeholder." In America, we would bring on
board some patients, two nurses, a few lawyers, a male and
female psychiatrist perhaps, a cardiologist, an orthopedist,
and maybe an executive from Pfizer. Also, we would need a
few hospital administrators and some insurance people—for
health insurance, medical malpractice, and workers compensation. A device executive who makes orthopedic screws and
artificial joints might be helpful, and maybe even a sales-

person for self-propelled wheelchairs. Their interests would all cancel out, and they would produce standards ensuring cost efficiency and excellent care. Right?

Forget it. This strategy created the current chaos. *Not one of these people should be at the table.* The only way this committee scheme might work would be to have *no conflicts of interest allowed.* We must not permit doctors, lawyers, industry representatives, or anyone else who makes a dime on healthcare to decide or advise about anything.

A group of academics, mathematicians on salary perhaps, might work. Medicine is easy for people like this to understand—they are smarter than physicians. They would know statistics better than a machinist and would hopefully have had fewer criminal settlements than Pfizer.

CHAPTER 37

YOUR PERSONAL
HEALTHCARE PHILOSOPHY

> *Medicine has become a pseudo-religion; our patients must be gently*
> *encouraged into apostasy and renunciation... [We have all] been*
> *enslaved by the medical–industrial complex, and it is time we*
> *rebelled. Society needs to reach a new accommodation with old age*
> *and death.*

> — SEAMUS O'MAHONY, *CAN MEDICINE BE CURED*
> (2019)

HERE IS THE SILVER LINING: when you better understand your
fragile life and the limitations of medicine, you will avoid
getting sucked into a lot of useless nonsense.

By 60, most people have some coronary artery disease; by
70, most have cancers growing somewhere. Nortin Hadler
states the cold facts: "Any claim to a science that offers a path
to longevity beyond eighty-five years is fatuous… over 85,
you are off-warranty." My pathologist friend Chris Gonzales
adds, "something will get you, eventually." He cuts up dead
people for a living, so he knows.

Worrying about your lifespan or expecting medicine to

save you will not bring you peace. Instead, focus on your mission and the tasks. Be philosophical about your health as it declines.

At the end of life, some people can become more grateful rather than more afraid because they have learned to treasure each moment. Max Ehrmann wrote, "Gracefully surrender the things of youth. Nurture strength of spirit to shield you in sudden misfortune."

My friend Dana understood this. He taught me what he could over his final year, and I loved him dearly. He had coronary artery disease with congestive heart failure, and for months, we knew he might die.

He had always been optimistic, but during this period, he ignored all negativity and told me he felt better and better. He knew he had no time for regrets, complaints, whining, or worry. I realized later that we are in the same position as Dana every day of our lives.

The following works. How you feel is the best measure of your health, not some lab test. Your diet, exercise, and sleep habits are more important than any pill or procedure.

Long life is more likely with good luck, good genetics, peace of mind, and drug avoidance, including nicotine and alcohol. Healthy relationships are essential, but medical care most often is not.

Most aches and pains go away on their own. Ignore them unless they are persistent.

The following does not work. Over half of prescribed drugs are useless, nearly useless, or bad for you. If medications are not working, look for alternatives. There are no side effects for drugs you do not take.

When you have no symptoms, avoid looking for fresh troubles with scans and lab tests. Preventive care is ineffective. You lose time, money, and tranquility, and it could subject you to more testing or some treatment nightmare.

Nortin Hadler said, "To restate the mantra, one never wants to submit to screening unless the test is accurate, the disease is important, and we can do something about it."

For the elderly, most medical care is ineffective. Since the end is approaching, a cure for one condition is unlikely to extend life. Dignity, comfort, and practical support should be the goals. Refusing invasive procedures and medications is usually best. In 180 AD, Marcus Aurelius wrote: "Dying is a part of life, and like everything else, it should be done to the best of your abilities[1]."

If you accept a diagnosis, you may persuade yourself to throw away your decision-making and become dependent on providers. For example, think twice before believing you need medicine for sleep, depression, or cholesterol. Think twice before you consider back surgery when your pain has only lasted a few months. None of these work very well.

Listen to opinions, make your decisions, and have no regrets. Most times, a doctor's only power is to name a problem, which is useless if there is no reasonable therapy. Running to them for everything damages your morale and finances. Healthcare decisions that seem essential often make little difference because the remedies are worthless.

How to work with physicians: They deserve your respect for their broad knowledge, experience, and training, but do not let them intimidate you. Real physicians still have much to offer, so do not abandon trust altogether. They are trying their best despite their confusion and conflicts of interest. The finest among them use art on the fringes of science, extending life, occasionally curing, and supporting us in our struggles. If you accept treatment, let them do the worrying for you. This is why you pay them.

Physicians believe in what they do—I still believe some of it—but this does not mean we are always right. The more dogmatic we are, the less you should trust us. If you do not understand what we say, we may not, either. Or perhaps we are selling you something unnecessary.

Research, insist on proof, and challenge everything. The more you learn about the limits of science, the more you realize that your gut reactions are sometimes better than expert opinions. You may lose nothing by saying no, so at each step, consider getting on with your life and taking your chances without medical care. It is your body, and you are in charge, so act like it.

Conclusions for patients: Some healthcare is useful, so you need to figure out what is best for you. Avoiding controversial treatments, surgeries, and medications will save you from much harm except for the collective expense, which we all shoulder together.

Greedy corporations are in control. Destroying them is impossible, unless, like Purdue, they have had a hand in murdering several hundred thousand people. The prosecutors permit the others to pay us off and continue their crimes. Since these businesses are almost untouchable, worrying about them is futile.

For peace of mind, we must each get a life and stop obsessing and gossiping about healthcare. None of the following people benefit from our meddling. Not our friend with prostate cancer, our auntie who saw the cardiologist recently, nor our mother in the nursing home.

Conclusions for physicians: We volunteered for this job, and our name is yet on medicine's door. Our power and integrity have dwindled—part has been taken from us, and part we gave away. But as captains of this ship, we must accept all blame and shoulder all responsibility.

We still have much to give and a doctor's role can be transcendent. The best of us are mentors, counselors, and at the end of life, some of us function as priests. Our promise is to spend what strength and skill and heart that we have in the service of others. When we forget this, we are lost.

If we can rise anew as leaders, we may justify what trust remains in us. No one else can do the job, and our home is being torched around us by the dragons lodging in our basement. They have been eating our children, and it must stop.

CHAPTER 38

WHAT HAPPENED TO MY COLLEAGUES AND ME?

In the midst of winter, I found there was, within me, an invincible summer.

— ALBERT CAMUS

BACK TO MY PERSONAL STORY. The family of the patient who died of the lidocaine overdose sued us, and after several agonizing years, our insurance company settled. The family of the woman with the fat embolus never sued because they had no chance of winning. It was an unpreventable risk of the procedure. Because I had two deaths, the California medical board looked at it. Like the vast majority of cases, they negotiated it to a probation. I still had my license, but they required me to have ten percent of my patient records reviewed. I attended a few days of testing.

Dr. Gøtzsche had touched the "third rail of healthcare," vaccines. He pointed out that the corporations had hidden half of the Human Papilloma Virus studies, just like they did with the antidepressants. As a result, the Cochrane collaboration had an excuse to remove him from their board. It was a minority vote, considering the abstentions. This was a disaster for Cochrane's reputation, and many observers thought the industry's money was behind it.

He explained the situation in a book, a blog article, and an explanatory document. Without his guidance, the Cochrane has lost much credibility and good karma. Maryanne Demasi, PhD, in the *BMJ*, said they were "a sinking ship."

Abraham Katz became very discouraged after Cochrane kicked Dr. Gøtzsche out. He wrote:

The media have been saying that Gøtzsche had significant conflicts of interest, his calculations regarding the HPV vaccine were wrong, and that he was a lunatic who is controversial just for the sake of it. They ignored that a third of the HPV panel at Cochrane resigned in protest after his ouster.

The Japanese Ministry of Health withdrew their recommendation for the vaccine as well. The percent receiving it went from 80% to 1%. This country has an excellent system to report harm from drugs. They found that the HPV vaccine had three times the adverse events of any vaccine that they had ever used. If a highly educated country like Japan can conclude that this treatment was unsafe, then I would expect the Cochrane report to find, in their customary fashion, that not enough high-quality studies have been done to determine the truth. This is what they offer most of the time.

I am now doubtful that we can trust the Cochrane Collaboration. My skepticism started in 2016, when they claimed, contrary to the data, that tPA was effective in reducing stroke symptoms. One of their committees, loaded with industry influences, supported this expensive clot-dissolving treatment. This contradicted their opinion a few years earlier when they said it did not work. Cochrane was one of the last respected refuges of quality science. When there wasn't enough evidence to make a statement, they were always willing to say that the answer was unclear instead of guessing.

These events are a debacle. I am concerned that medicine is moving in the wrong direction, which is tragic.

Nortin Hadler has spent the best part of three decades trying to get his ideas across to physicians and legislators. I doubt it has been easy. He has a beautiful body of work in his books, blogs, and YouTube presentations.

Wendy Dolin, who won the $3 million judgment after her husband's (generic) Paxil-related suicide, lost her appeal. The issue was whether the original patent holder's concealment of complications and deaths during the approval process made them responsible for other deaths caused later by generics. If her lawyers had won, the original manufacturer might have been on the hook for hundreds of millions of dollars.

Wendy has not let the appeals court defeat her; she was not suing to make money but to get the word out. She has continued to work on her awareness group about drug-related suicides. Her annual event in the fall of 2019 was a success.

I speak to Martha Rosenberg frequently, and we support each other.

My biggest personal gut-punch was when I found out how industry propaganda had overrun the Internet, including social media. The disease-mongering discouraged me the most. I saw an obviously ghostwritten article "How Pharma Sales Reps Help Me Be a More Up-to-Date Doctor." The ubiquity of these messages affected me more than the other swindles.

I continued my cosmetic surgery practice on a small scale through the fall of 2019. I liked the patient interactions and was the master of a few specialized surgeries such as liposuction, fat transplantation, and breast augmentation through the navel. I finally retired when I was sixty-six.

I continue to learn. I read about other government-supported industries: defense, energy, and arguably the worst, banking. Just like healthcare, they are corrupted by outside funding, special status, and tax advantages.

I also contemplate the fiercely competitive corporate

sectors that have been such a boon to us all—hotels, airlines, computers, and rental cars. Corporations, even whole industries, have personalities. Some are wonderful, and some are criminals.

I wonder about the rest of science. Is it as shaky, biased, and degraded by money as medicine?

CHAPTER 39

APPENDIX: NATIONAL ACTION PLAN

✪ DEFINE the following unethical actions as crimes and prosecute them aggressively: disease-mongering, advertising lies, and promotion of scientific misconduct.

✪ Criminalize concealment and distortion in the medical literature.

✪ Preserve all studies online, both the failures and successes, along with complete data. Since our public funds pay these companies, we must change the laws so the public, not they, owns all drug and medical product information.

✪ Prosecute conflicts of interest as criminal acts the same way we do insider dealing in financial markets.

✪ Define gifts and sponsorship as bribery and prosecute the corporations doing this.

✪ Eliminate fee-for-service.

✪ Criminalize the use of public money for healthcare lobbying and medical advertising.

✪ Give the money to entities similar to Kaiser Permanente. We must base funding on actuarial healthcare costs per year of life. Money for individual procedures, hospital stay-days, or any other itemized care rewards misuse.

✪ Get rid of bad therapies. To start, we must model other

countries' more conservative, less wasteful standards. The goal is to incrementally defund mammograms, angioplasty, CABG surgery, routine colonoscopy, parts of orthopedics, most of psychiatry, and a lot more.

○ Abolish healthcare patents.

○ Take most drugs off prescription and make them over-the-counter. Restrict the use of all psychiatric drugs and antibiotics by making them schedule II just like the opioids and amphetamines.

○ Strip corporations of any plaintiffs protection that goes along with the FDA patent process.

○ Develop this plan using people with no conflicts of interest. We must not permit doctors, lawyers, industry repre-sentatives, or anyone else who makes a dime on healthcare to decide or advise about anything. A group of academics, math-ematicians on salary perhaps, might work.

RESOURCES

Hundreds of books were published in the last few decades related to medical corruption. Many contain naïve, wishful thinking, or boorishly irritate the reader with political cate-chisms. They nearly all have too much respect for physicians and healthcare.

Everyone has biases. Doctors want to be doctors, and pharmacists want to sell drugs for insurance payment or to sell supplements without oversight. Even the whistleblower Peter Rost has a hard time utterly condemning his former drug company employers. When I spoke to my gynecologist friend regarding hysterectomies, he said, "Don't go there." Retired journal editors are fond of their former employers. Psychiatric technicians saw so many people brain-damaged by medications that they cannot conceive that the drugs might be a benefit for anyone, even very sick people.

Some books describe history. For example, there are

descriptions of Medicare's Byzantine, Sovietesque structure, and perverse incentives, as if that ship had not already run into an iceberg and sunk.

Many said I was opening a can of worms with my work. What I found was a dumpster of worms, and I finally realized that I could only examine what was squirming on the surface. Studying orthopedic, oncologic, and cardiac academics could have taken years. It went on and on. I wrote this book—but the book also wrote me. It destroyed my illusions painfully.

For the books that influenced me the most, please visit DrYohoAuthor.com.

The best Internet sources are the following. None is perfect.

The *Cochrane Collaboration* evaluates healthcare topics using 37,000 independent contributors from 130 countries. Their meta-analyses dissect and amalgamate the best studies. They have a better reputation than any journal and take no commercial funding. They are not perfect: they still have to work with industry-sponsored research.

TheNNT.com (NNT=Number needed to treat) has brief summaries about many healthcare issues. These are complete, easy to understand, and address hundreds of topics. They accept no outside funding or advertisements. It is an excellent effort, but they examine the same imperfect data source as the Cochrane. You do not have to be a doctor to comprehend this material.

Worstpills.org: Sidney Wolfe, the founder, is a prominent member of Ralph Nader's *Public Citizen*, and has campaigned against the use of many ineffective medications. This group recommends waiting seven years after drugs go on the market before using them because their problems usually get sorted out by then.

ProPublica.org tracks an individual physician's Medicare income.

For akathisia: This is a severe drug-related restlessness sometimes associated with suicide and violence. For information and support groups, see the following websites. Brace yourself—this is difficult reading. As you scan it, recall Martha Rosenberg's question: Were there reports of older women biting their friends to death, preteen girls hanging themselves, or mothers drowning their own babies before the SSRI epidemic?

Some non-psychiatric medications given for allergy, epilepsy, nausea, pain, and PMS are chemical relatives of psychiatric drugs and have identical side effects. I met a woman at a conference who took a few months of Reglan for heartburn. She subsequently had akathisia symptoms and felt like killing herself for over three years. She learned that the drug was a phenothiazine (neuroleptic) like Thorazine.

✪ *SSRIstories.org*: 5000 news reports of suicide, murder, and other violence related to the SSRIs.

✪ Wendy Dolin's "Medication-Induced Suicide Prevention and Education Foundation in Memory of Stewart Dolin" (MISSD) group's purpose is to raise awareness of akathisia.

She formed it after the events described in the Welcome to Big Industry chapter. She says:

> *Our mission is to increase awareness of the side effects, including severe ones such as akathisia that occur when medication dosage is stopped or changed. What the drug companies have tried to hide about akathisia is that it gives ordinary people suicidal thoughts. During my trial, Dr. Healy explained this to the jury, and they saw the numbers of people who died during the drug trials. I think that's what won our case.*

Ms. Dolin produced a cartoon video presentation with a simple explanation of the syndrome.

✪ *Woodymatters.com* was developed by the wife of a man who killed himself after taking an SSRI. It tells the story.

⊘ *Prescription Suicide?* A documentary film about the SSRI drug tragedies occurring when children take them.

For networking: the *Lown Institute* is a nationwide group of professionals who are well-informed about these issues. Networking with them was a pleasure for me at their 2018 DC meeting.

For patient medical information, the best sites are *mayoclinic.org.* and Wikipedia. Stay away from *webmd.com* and its relatives. They are heavily industry-funded.

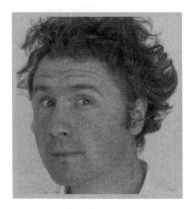

Ben Goldacre

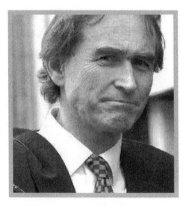

David Healy

STAY IN TOUCH

I hope we now have a relationship. I am distributing this book free for a limited time at this LINK. If you do not understand e-books, the support people there will help you download an app and start reading. If you haven't discovered Kindle or other ebook readers, you will find they are the easiest way to read—anything—and handily access references. Here is my website: DrYohoAuthor.com. Click this LINK to read other reviews on my Amazon site. Buy the book in any format HERE.

If you think my work is valuable, I have a few favors to ask, in order of importance.

1) Use this link to gift this book to your friends, or better, your entire list.

2) Please make time to write an Amazon review. I will read it, and I appreciate you for doing it. Reviewing a book before finishing it is acceptable. You can update what you say later if you want. Click this LINK to get straight to the reviews.

3) Optional: donate to my gofundme.com account HERE. I will use the money to educate others.

I answer all polite questions at DrYohoauthor@gmail.com. Email if you want me to speak to your group. Mailing address: 99 West California Blvd #50007, Pasadena, CA, 91115

For my (former) cosmetic surgery career, see DrYoho.com and Facebook

FELLOW TRAVELERS WHO
AIDED ME

Friends and acquaintances are the surest paths to fortune.

— Arthur Schopenhauer (1788-1860)

The following people helped me with suggestions, proofreading, and ideas: James Bolton, PhD, Phil Horner, JD, Joe Liberty, Tony Mangubat, MD, Denis Portero, JD, Pharm D, Russell Robinson, and George Tuttle, MD.

Lynne Bateson is a professional writer and friend who was supportive and encouraging. She took the time to rewrite some sections. Some of the best writing here is hers.

Michael Bellomo is a full-time writer and my literary mentor. He liked my content and encouraged me to develop a 'voice.' His major work these days is paranormal romance fiction, but he has written nine books on nonfiction medical subjects. He gave me many writing tips and did not realize how closely I listened to him.

Mark Berman, MD, did a complete read-through at several stages and was encouraging. His respected opinion kept me going through many nay-sayers.

Neal Handel, MD, wrote a letter to me after reviewing an early draft. His encouragement meant a lot.

George Boris, MD, read early drafts and was flattering about the content even before editing improved it. He already knew that much of medicine was ineffective.

Jeff Brown told me he understood my prose better than other writers at a point when I was not sure about the project.

Bruce Chisholm, MD, taught me many things. He advised me many years ago that antidepressants were no good. He understood they were ineffective long before I saw the data.

Robin Dorfman is a top editor who immediately spotted issues others had missed.

James Friederich, Ph.D., is an academic psychologist, statistician, and dear friend who read early drafts of this manuscript and took it seriously. We wrestled at Oberlin College together, and he taught me a lot then and now.

Nortin Hadler, MD, generously read the chapters about medical statistics and coronary disease and encouraged me at an early phase. He is a top medical intellectual, the kind who speaks at graduation ceremonies.

Wendy Dolin's story began when her husband killed himself after he took generic Paxil for a week. Wendy is a super-networker and introduced me to her group devoted to educating people about drugs that cause suicide.

Sue Kientz is a Caltech administrator who took time away from dealing with the wild characters over there to do a first-round edit.

Herb Laeger, PhD, is my climbing buddy and a laser physicist. He spent many hours correcting and improving both my concepts and my prose. I knew he was a brilliant guy but learned he also had writing skills.

Tom Lane is a professional editor who read the manuscript twice. It amazed me how much he knew about the subjects and how much more he grasped with this brief exposure. I reorganized the entire thing on his advice.

Jeanne Lenzer was kind enough to review the book and correct some errors.

Tucker Max told me not to hesitate to take another six months to complete the project at a point when I thought I was nearly done. I took over another year. At his seminar, he encouraged me about the importance of the subject.

Martha Rosenberg: After stalking her online for months, I finally met her. She has been studying the FDA for decades and knows medical and regulatory corruption well. She has become a friend.

Neal Rouzier, MD, had many doubts but was my original inspiration.

Kyle Scott took my book on as a serious project, and let me know his reactions in granular detail. He informed my thinking about how a top-flight reader reacts to my prose and thought processes.

Jeff Segal, MD, JD, read the book through sophisticated eyes and made many helpful suggestions.

Peter Gøtzsche kindly encouraged me at an early stage. He helped found the Cochrane Collaboration, the world's most respected medical analysis group, and was head of the Danish division until 2018. He is a giant, the best we have.

Héctor Tobar, who shares a Pulitzer for his reporting of the Los Angeles riots, laughed at the idea I could complete a book in a year. He has several bestsellers, each of which took at least three years.

Becca B. Jenkins is one of the best creative and structural writers of any of these brilliant people. She reorganized some sections.

Sheila Buff knows more medicine than 95 percent of physicians. She worked through the complete manuscript and corrected some of my misconceptions and misstatements.

Mira de Vries was generous with her time and criticism. I cannot thank her enough.

Leiah Cooper came in at the terminal writing stages and

encouraged me by her rapid acquisition of all the major concepts despite having little medical background. Either she is a genius, or by then, my explanations were credible, or both. As she learned, her outrage and her active mind propelled her to generously fact-check and update references for the bulk of the work. I clarified several sections as I watched her reactions. If Leiah did not understand the material, who could? She helped put the manuscript into the proper format for publication, which is indispensable for readability.

Brian Dobrin, JD, proved to be one of my most literate and critical readers. He saw logical and phrasing issues that made it past over thirty others.

Steven Browne is a professional songwriter who produces his own music. He was a fantastic audio advisor and editor.

Grant Horner, PhD, is my climbing buddy and a Milton scholar with several scholarly books and many articles in print. He taught college composition for 26 years and knows six languages. He was kind enough to read the book for stylistic issues.

My wife, Judy Yoho, thought this book was a fool's errand from the start but has been supportive as always. I tell her every day: thank you for everything!

NOTES

8. Disease-Mongering & Bogus Cures

1. **For more about Avandia,** see *drugwatch.com*, the *BMJ*, the *New England Journal of Medicine*, and Peter Gøtzsche's book, *Deadly Medicine and Organised Crime*.

9. Pharma's Marketing And Bullying

1. Duff Wilson's article (*NY Times*, 2011) explains.
2. See Gardiner Harris's NY Times article, 2009

11. Opioids And "Pain Management"

1. Smith told his sad story on Medium.com and also has a podcast.

17. Prozac And Relatives

1. For much more about this violence than most readers can stomach, see Deadly Psychiatry and Organized Denial (2015) by Peter Gøtzsche.
2. May 25th, 1984 communication to Lilly US from Lilly Bad Homburg

18. Antipsychotics Are Disastrous

1. For many other anecdotes, see Whitaker's *MadInAmerica.com* blog.

22. Easy Math Explains Everything

1. This idea was from Vinay Prasad and Adam Cifu's *Ending Medical Reversal* (2015) and also Vinay Prasad's *Malignant* (2020).

25. Science Debunked The Heart Doctors

1. David Newman's 2014 review of CABG in theNNT.com is a balanced commentary from a time when the literature was already mature. He cites two dozen key references.
2. *TheNNT.com* has an excellent summary.

26. Surgery: Money Before Patients

1. *Crooked: Outwitting the Back Pain Industry, 2017.*
2. *Stabbed in the Back, 2009.*

27. Screening Tests Are Useless

1. *Hippocrates' Shadow* (2008) by David Newman and a comprehensive 2013 *NY Times* review by Peggy Orenstein both agree.
2. US National Cancer Institute
3. Tampa Bay Times and The Center for Investigative Reporting

28. Failed Cancer Treatments

1. National Cancer Institute
2. Gilbert Welch, MD, described the debacle in the *NEJM* (2014).
3. National Cancer Institute
4. Much of this material came from dermatologist David Epstein's online blog and a 2017 *NY Times* exposé of dermatology by Katie Hafner and Griffin Palmer.

29. Futile Cpr And Overprescribing

1. A literature review by David Newman in *TheNNT.com* from 2010 confirmed that ACLS medicines do not save lives. For more, see his book *Hippocrates Shadow* (2008).

30. Billing Scams & Specialty Warfare

1. Deborah Sullivan reported this tacky rivalry as far back as 2001 in *Cosmetic Surgery: The Cutting Edge of Commercial Medicine in America.*

32. Hospitals Are Sharks

1. Elisabeth Rosenthal's book, *An American Sickness*, Steven Brill's book *Bitter Pill*, and his *Time* magazine articles are the best descriptions of hospitals and the rest of the expense side of medicine. See also Elisabeth Rosenthal's articles on the Kaiser Permanente website, including one about bills that should be defined as fraud but are legal. Much of the material from this chapter came from these excellent and readable sources.

35. Legislative Sausage-Making

1. For more about this, Google "EMR fiasco." Dozens of articles appear with "fiasco" in the title.

36. Save Our Nation

1. See Martha Rosenberg's book and *drugwatch.com* for supporting material.

37. Your Personal Healthcare Philosophy

1. *Meditations*, Marcus Aurelius

ABOUT THE AUTHOR

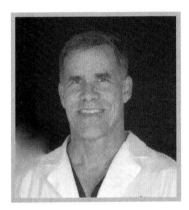

Robert Yoho, MD. (2010)

Dr. Yoho is 66 years old in 2020. He spent three decades as a cosmetic surgeon after a career as an emergency physician. His generalist training gives him perspective and allows him to avoid favoring any medical specialty.

He has had little dealings with hospitals, big Pharma, or insurance companies before he wrote this book. No one has ever considered him a "whale" prescriber or device implanter. He retired from medical practice in 2019.

ABBREVIATED PROFESSIONAL CV:

❂ American Society of Cosmetic Breast Surgery: fellow, trustee, officer, and past-president.

❂ American Board of Cosmetic Surgery: passed board exams and twice re-certified.

✪ American Board of Emergency Medicine: passed board exams and twice re-certified.

✪ Fellow, American Academy of Cosmetic Surgery (inactive).

✪ New Body Cosmetic Surgery Center: founder & director (inactive).

✪ American Association Ambulatory Health Care (AAAHC) accredited surgical/medical practice for over 25 years.

ABBREVIATED CLIMBER CV:

✪ El Capitan, Half Dome (Yosemite): 24-hour ascents
✪ Free ascents of Astroman (11.c) and Crucifix (12.a)
✪ First ascents in Yosemite, Joshua Tree, Devils Tower
✪ Solo ascents to 5.10c

ALSO BY ROBERT YOHO, MD

✪ *A New Body in One Day* (2004)

✪ *Butchered By Big Pharma* (pending pub)

✪ *Butchered By Big Food* (pending pub)

✪ Twenty articles in medical journals.

✪ COSMETIC SURGERY WEBSITE: DrYoho.com

✪ AUTHOR WEBSITE: DrYohoAuthor.com

Made in the USA
Columbia, SC
24 September 2020

21312294R00212